VITILIGO – MANAGEMENT AND THERAPY

Edited by **Kelly KyungHwa Park**
and **Jenny Eileen Murase**

Vitiligo – Management and Therapy
Edited by Kelly KyungHwa Park and Jenny Eileen Murase

Published by InTech
Janeza Trdine 9, 51000 Rijeka, Croatia

Publishing Process Manager Anja Filipovic

Technical Editor Teodora Smiljanic

Cover Designer InTech Design Team

Additional hard copies can be obtained from orders@intechopen.com

Vitiligo – Management and Therapy, Edited by Kelly KyungHwa Park
and Jenny Eileen Murase
p. cm.
ISBN 978-953-307-731-4

For EU product safety concerns:
IN TECH d.o.o., Prolaz Marije Krucifikse Kozulić 3, 51000 Rijeka, Croatia,
info@intechopen.com or visit our website at intechopen.com.

Meet the editors

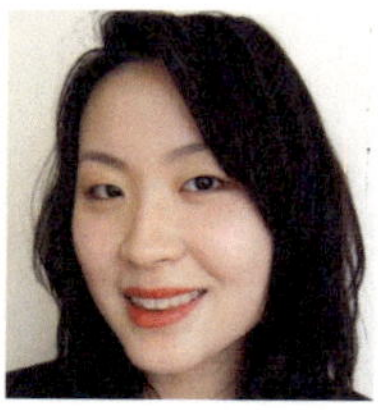

Dr. Kelly KyungHwa Park, M.D. is the Clinical Research and Phototherapy Fellow at the Department of Dermatology of the University of California, San Francisco. Dr. Park graduated from the accelerated Bachelor of Science and Doctor of Medicine (B.S./M.D.) program at the University of Akron and the Northeast Ohio Medical University, where she also earned her Certificate in Bioethics. As an undergraduate, she was on the Dean's List and completed a double major in Natural Sciences and History and a minor in Chemistry. During medical school, she was selected for the Weill Medical College of Cornell University Travelers Summer Research Fellowship Program and the Memorial Sloan-Kettering Cancer Center Medical Student Summer Fellowship Program. She subsequently completed her internship in Internal Medicine at St. Vincent's Hospital Manhattan. Dr. Park has authored numerous peer-reviewed manuscripts for such publications as the Journal of the American Academy of Dermatology, Archives of Dermatology, and the British Medical Journal.

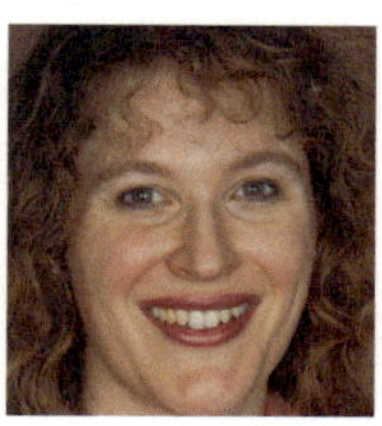

Dr. Jenny Eileen Murase is an Assistant Clinical Professor of Dermatology at the University of California, San Francisco, and the Director of Phototherapy for the Palo Alto Foundation Medical Group. Dr. Murase received her medical degree from the University of California, Irvine; she received the Dean's award and was the first graduate with distinction in clinical research. Board certified in dermatology, she is currently the editor of the Women's Dermatologic Society. Active in clinical research and teaching, she was voted by the UCSF dermatology residents best dermatology instructor among the adjunct clinical faculty in 2010. Course director at the American Academy of Dermatology Annual meeting the past four years, she serves on the AAD Needs Assessment and Educational Program Evaluation Committee Task Force and the Professional Expert Evaluation Review Program. Dr. Murase has coauthored more than 40 peer-reviewed book chapters and articles, and actively reviews for five major dermatology journals.

Contents

Preface

Vitiligo is a common yet frequently misunderstood disease. Despite the historical and cultural significance of vitiligo, as well as its impact on the lives of those affected, the pathogenesis, clinical presentation, and management of vitiligo remains elusive. The expertise and knowledge of an international group of experts and clinicians well-versed in vitiligo have been gathered to provide the reader with a practical guide to vitiligo.

We hope that the reader can gain insight into vitiligo as a disease and its management, as well as demonstrate the ability to apply the fundamental concepts covered in this book. Our wish is that this book will be a concise yet comprehensive tool for the dissemination of the newest developments and therapeutic advances in vitiligo.

Acknowledgements

I am grateful for the unwavering support of my co-editor and mentor, Jenny Murase, M.D., as well as my mentors, John Koo, M.D., and Rebecca Tung, M.D.

As always, I am thankful to my parents, Youn Wook Park, M.D., and Kay KongBum Shin-Park, Ph.D., my sister Sonja Park, M.A., and Edgar, for their endless encouragement.

I also wish to acknowledge the nurses and staff at the University of California San Francisco, Psoriasis and Skin Treatment Center, who make every day pleasant for physicians and patients alike.

Kelly KyungHwa Park, MD
Department of Dermatology
University of California San Francisco
San Francisco, California
USA

To my Katsuyuki, Emi, Lilia, and Kento for reminding me of the richness of life and the joy of laughter, and to my parents for teaching me how to give to others: for nothing is more important than family!

Jenny Eileen Murase, MD
Palo Alto Foundation Medical Group
Department of Dermatology
Mountain View, California
USA

Introductory Chapter

An Illustrated Guide to Clinical Vitiligo with Expert Opinion

Kelly KyungHwa Park[1] and Seung-Kyung Hann[2]
[1]*University of California San Francisco Department of Dermatology, San Francisco, California*
[2]*Drs. Woo & Hann Skin Center, Korea Institute of Vitiligo Research, Seoul*
[1]*USA*
[2]*Korea*

1. Introduction

Vitiligo is an idiopathic disorder of depigmentation that can be both disfiguring and distressing. It is essential to optimize one's approach to the vitiligo patient, which is dependent on a working knowledge of this common condition, because vitiligo can show various clinical patterns with unpredictable courses. This requires recognition of the various patterns of disease as well as clinical presentation. Furthermore, this will guide accurate clinical diagnosis and bring with it the ability to distinguish vitiligo from other pigmentary disorders. Awareness of both the common and potentially serious comorbidities associated with vitiligo will determine whether a multidisciplinary approach to care is appropriate. The concerns of special patient populations with vitiligo should be acknowledged. An appreciation of the psychosocial effects of vitiligo is also a necessary part of understanding vitiligo patients.

2. Clinical presentation

Vitiligo affects an estimated 0.5-1% of the global population, with similar incidence rates found in males and females without racial, ethnic, or geographic predilection (Halder, 1997; Silverberg & Travis, 2006). Half of all vitiligo patients present before the age of 20, however, it can appear at almost any age (Halder, 1997; Silverberg & Travis, 2006). The natural history of vitiligo is insidious, and prognosis is generally unknown. It is characterized by the appearance of white or chalky-white amelanotic macules or patches. Typically, one or more discrete round, oval, or linear macules of varying sizes are found. In some cases, lesions may be circumscribed by a mildly erythematous border, which is indicative of an inflammatory process. The disease tends to progress with age in a symmetrical, centrifugal pattern, and can follow a rapid or protracted time course. Lesions can be distinguished by Wood's lamp examination or made more apparent by tanning of surrounding normal skin. Vitiligo is usually asymptomatic, although pruritus may be reported, particularly when lesions are spreading.

Vitiligo can appear anywhere on the body and mucous membranes. The face, dorsal hands, intertriginous areas, umbilicus, sacrum, and anogenitial regions are most commonly affected. The Koebner phenomenon is associated with vitiligo; areas of repeated trauma, friction, or chronic contact are common sites of involvement. Other inciting factors include mental stress, surgery, pregnancy, and sunburn (Esposito-Smythers, *et al.*, 2010).

Leukotrichia (depigmented hairs) of the body is common, and seen in at least 10% to over 60% of patients (Ortonne JP, 2008). Poliosis presents as localized patches (usually isolated) of white or gray hair, and is frequently observed with vitiligo of the scalp.

3. Classification & patterns

Vitiligo can be divided into types which can further be described by distribution, location, and other characteristics. However, the classification of vitiligo is complex and much debated. Multiple terminologies are used to describe vitiligo, and often several descriptions are used to describe one vitiligo entity. A basic "glossary" of vitiligo is presented below in order to help distinguish common terms seen in the literature, despite a current lack of consensus of some terminology (Table 1). These classifications will be described below, with supporting detail reflecting the views of international vitiligo consensus experts.

The main types of vitiligo are **non-segmental vitiligo** (**NSV**, also referred to as generalized vitiligo, common vitiligo, and historically as vitiligo vulgaris), and **segmental vitiligo** (**SV**, "asymmetric vitiligo"). NSV can present as focal disease, confined to the mucous membranes, appear in an acrofacial distribution, or be generalized or universal. SV generally refers to disease occurring in a zosteriform, dermatomal, or Blaschko's distribution, which can be focal or in rare cases, be found on mucosal surfaces. It is also useful to describe of the segments pattern by number of segments involved: unilateral, bilateral, or mixed.

NSV was originally classified by Lerner as generalized vitiligo, and there is growing support for restoration of this term (Lerner, 1959). South American vitiligo experts insist that segmental vitiligo should be referred to as unilateral vitiligo and that non-segmental should be bilateral vitiligo. However, this concept of classification is not accepted by the whole international vitiligo consensus group. NSV and SV are thought to differ in pathogenesis, which is substantiated by differences in presentation and associations. NSV is thought to be systemic in nature and occurs due to autoimmune-related melanocyte dysfunction, and although Koga first proposed that SV may be due to cutaneous sympathetic nerve dysfunction, the current accepted concept raised by Taïeb is that SV is the possible expression of cutaneous somatic mosaicism (Koga, 1977; Taïeb, *et al.*, 2008). Furthermore, an autoimmune mechanism may be involved in the early stages of SV, and from Hann's clinical experience, oral steroids may help during this time.

There is also a disputed "**unclassified**" or **mixed vitiligo** (**MV**) type that presents with features of both NSV and SV. It is sometimes used to describe those situations in which longer disease duration is required for evolution of disease into a definitive type (*i.e.*, NSV, SV) and subsequent accurate clinical diagnosis. MV was initially proposed by Hann and formally described by Taïeb and Picardo (Lee SJ, 2007). Spritz does not support this concept due to the very rare possibility of coincidental concurrence of both vitiligo types. As such, the unclassified or MV type is not recognized by most vitiligo experts.

Classification	Description	Common Locations	Notes
Nonsegmental Vitiligo/Generalized Vitiligo (common vitiligo, vitiligo vulgaris)	Wide distribution of nearly symmetrical typical amelanotic macules that are usually progressive	Fingers, volar wrists, mouth, eyes, groin and genitalia, axillae	Most common, >90% of cases
Segmental vitiligo (asymmetric vitiligo, unilateral or rarely, bilateral)	Depigmented patches confined to a predictable area of involvement	Dermatomal or semi-dermatomal pattern, or along Blaschko's lines	Early age of onset (childhood); no association with autoimmune or thyroid disease; >50% of those affected have poliosis
Mixed vitiligo	Combination of segmental vitiligo and nonsegmental vitiligo	Various	Proposed new vitiligo classification; segmental vitiligo can be severe
Focal vitiligo	Localized, solitary depigmented macule(s)	Face, neck, trunk	Most common in children
Acrofacial vitiligo	Localized patches	Distal fingertips and perioral regions	May involve mucous membranes
Universal vitiligo	Extensive disease with majority of the body involved	Up to entire body surface area	May be associated with Vogt-Koyanagi- Harada syndrome
Mucosal vitiligo	Typical macules of vitiligo	Mucous membranes	More apparent on darker skin types; disease is often refractory

Table 1. Glossary of Vitiligo

3.1 Non-segmental vitiligo

NSV can occur at any age and generally has a later age of onset than SV. It often suddenly appears and is usually progressive, with waxing and waning of disease. Periods of dormancy can last for many years and exacerbation of disease activity may last more than 12 months. Spontaneous incomplete repigmentation is at times reported by patients and is correlated with sun exposure (Passeron T, 2010).

Up to 50-75% of patients with focal disease will develop NSV (Liu, *et al.*, 2005; Passeron T, 2010). The extremities (*i.e.*, fingers and hands) and face are the most commonly reported initial sites of disease, while the extensor areas of the extremities are most commonly affected. There is also reported involvement of the malleoli, umbilicus, wrists, anterior tibial region, genitalia, axillae, and periorificial and periungual regions. Leukotrichia occurs in the late stages of disease (Ezzedine, *et al.*, 2011). Vitiligo is not usually accompanied with symptoms and signs of inflammation (Ezzedine, *et al.*, 2011). However, Ezzedine *et al* reported that NSV is more frequently preceded by pruritus compared with SV, especially prior to disease onset and flares. This is reported by 20% of NSV patients, a rate that is three times more than found in SV (Ezzedine, *et al.*, 2011). The Koebner phenomenon and halo nevi are more commonly associated with NSV than SV (Figure 1) (Taïeb & Picardo, 2009).

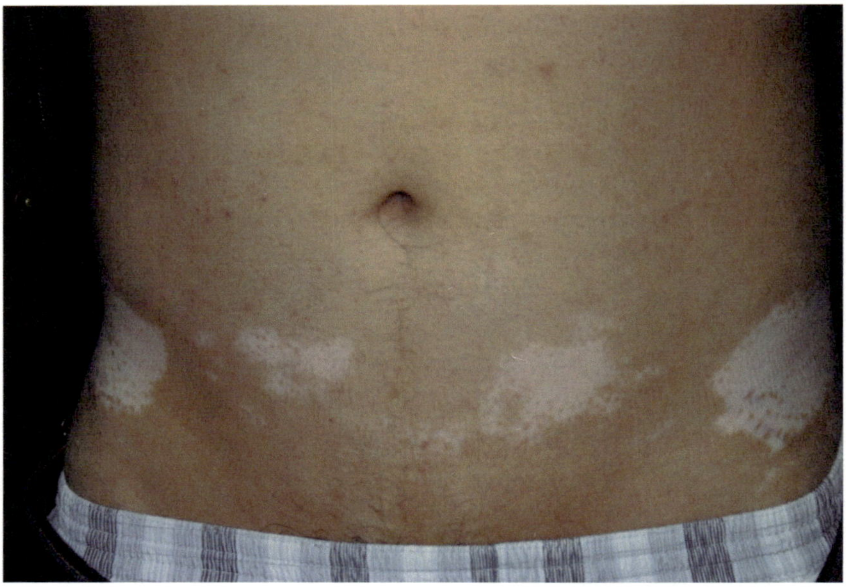

Fig. 1. The Koebner phenomenon is associated with vitiligo. This isomorphic phenomenon appears in this case due to clothing-related friction with resulting vitiligo lesions.

Concurrent autoimmune disease, in particular, thyroid dysfunction, is common in NSV patients and there is often a family history of autoimmune disease or vitiligo (Ezzedine, *et al.*, 2011; Taïeb & Picardo, 2009). It has been reported that familial vitiligo is a predictor of higher risk for NSV than SV, along with widespread involvement of disease. Also in these particular patients, the extent of disease is related to the presence of disease triggers, leukotrichia, and mucous membrane involvement (Karelson, *et al.*, 2011).

3.1.1 Subtypes

There are several subtypes of NSV. *Vitiligo universalis* (VU) is the rarest presentation of vitiligo and represents the most severe and progressive form of NSV. Its evolution is typically symmetric and can be rapid or occur after a dormant stage of NSV. Hair of the affected areas is generally affected, and the mucosal areas can be involved. Uveitis and consequent blindness can be reported, as well as mild hearing loss. Patients may have spontaneous repigmentation in perifollicular regions that are sun-exposed, likely due to retained melanocytes. Autoimmune thyroiditis and alopecia areata have been reported to be most commonly associated with VU (Passeron & Ortonne, 2010). VU may also be associated with the Vogt-Koyanagi-Harada (VKH) syndrome, an inflammatory autoimmune disorder targeting melanocytes leading to auditory, ocular, neurologic, and cutaneous symptoms. These patients account for 1-5% of patients presenting to the vitiligo clinic, and have characteristic vitiligo, alopecia, and poliosis (Albert, *et al.*, 1983).

Inflammatory vitiligo is characterized by erythematous margins and at times, pruritus (Figure 2). The sites of where inflammation settles become amelanotic.

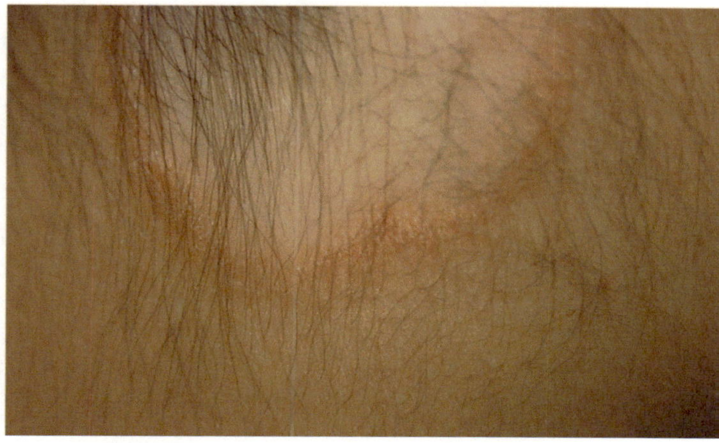

Fig. 2. Inflammatory vitiligo.

Blue vitiligo appears on sites of vitiligo resolution marked by postinflammatory hyperpigmentation, and from clinical observation, is only observed in darker skin types (Ivker, *et al.*, 1994).

Multichrome vitiligo is characterized by depigmentation coexisting with hypopigmented areas and normal skin color; this is most commonly seen in Fitzpatrick skin types IV-VI (Passeron T, 2010). *Trichrome vitiligo* shows an intermediate tan depigmentation between lesions of amelanosis and normal skin (Figure 3). *Quadrichrome vitiligo* has a dark brown

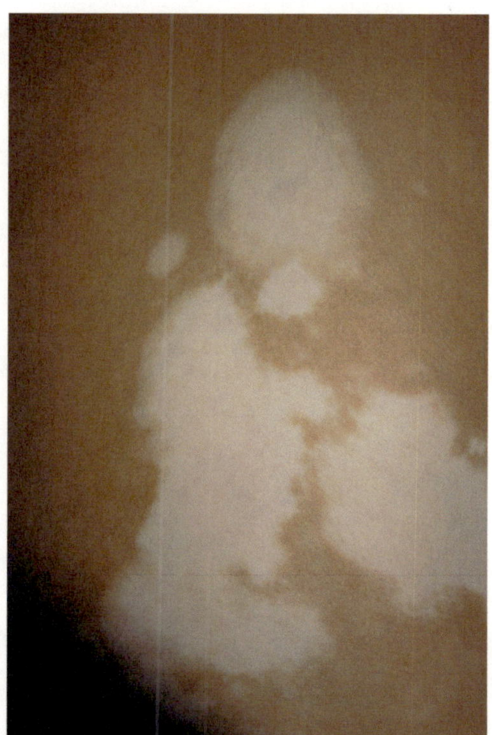

Fig. 3. Trichrome vitiligo

coloration at lesion margins or perifollicular areas. *Pentachrome* vitiligo includes the presence of a blue-gray area, totaling 5 shades. Trichrome, quadrichrome, and pentachrome vitiligo do not appear as a gradient of normal to amelanotic skin, but rather the appearance of specific shades of skin color that appear concurrently with typical amelanotic vitiligo. Histopathologic evidence suggests multichrome vitiligo can be a variant of active vitiligo (Hann, *et al.*, 2000).

Two controversial categories exist that are discussed for completeness:

Vitiligo ponctué consists of tiny, 1-2 mm confetti-like vitiliginous macules that may appear over areas of hyperpigmentation or over otherwise unaffected skin. This description may be inaccurate because this appearance may represent punctate leukoderma that can occur due to a number of etiologies.

Vitiligo minor appears as areas of homogenous depigmentation in Fitzpatrick skin types IV-VI (Passeron T, 2010). This classification is also debatable, although is described in major dermatology textbooks.

3.2 Segmental vitiligo

The prevalence of SV among individuals with vitiligo varies from 5–16.1% with 87% of cases occurring before the age of 30 (Park K, 1988; Song MS, 1994; Hann & Lee, 1996; Bang JS, 2000; Gauthier, *et al.*, 2003). In general, SV presents as a small (10-15 cm^2), elliptical depigmented patch that progresses in a typical pattern fairly quickly and ceases within a matter of days, months or years (Koga & Tango, 1988; Hann & Lee, 1996; Taïeb A, 2010; van Geel, *et al.*, 2011). This segmental pattern is not a general rule, but rather a guideline, as progression does not always follow a particular dermatome or Blaschkolinear pattern (van Geel, *et al.*, 2011). SV is most commonly found in a unilateral segmental pattern but can be very rarely distributed bilaterally (Figure 4), or progress to mixed vitiligo (van Geel, *et al.*, 2011). SV is usually dormant after expanding to involve a particular segment.

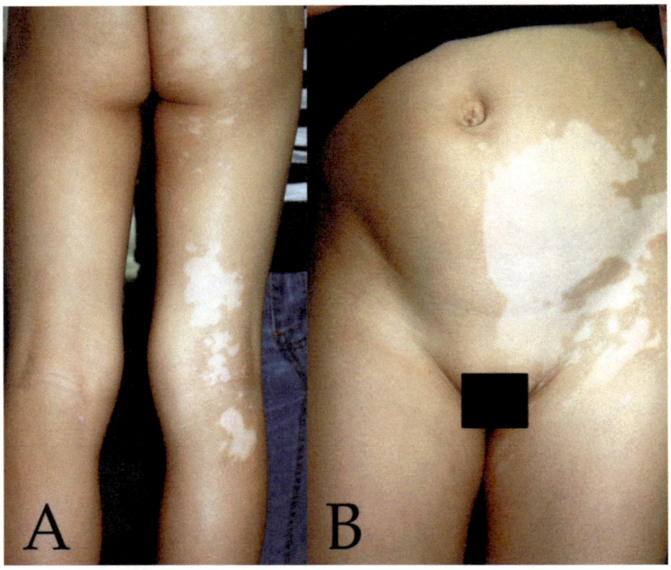

Fig. 4. Although rare, bilateral segmental vitiligo is a separate entity from nonsegmental vitiligo. A. A young female presents with involvement of the *right* posterior leg as well as, B. Involvement of the *left* torso

It is most common in childhood, and has no significant association with autoimmune disease. The majority of those affected have a single lesion, and presentation is most commonly of the face and head, followed by the trunk, limbs, extremities, and neck (Figures 5 and 6) (el-Mofty & el-Mofty, 1980; Barona, *et al.*, 1995; Hann & Lee, 1996; Hann, *et al.*, 1997; Bang JS, 2000). Leukotrichia and poliosis are common and rapidly progressive, occurring soon after SV onset (Taïeb & Picardo, 2009). This hair involvement complicates nearly 50%

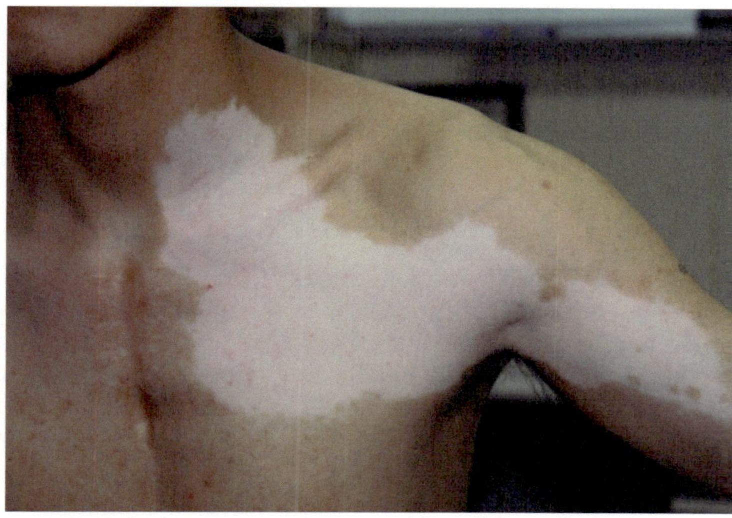

Fig. 5. Segmental vitiligo

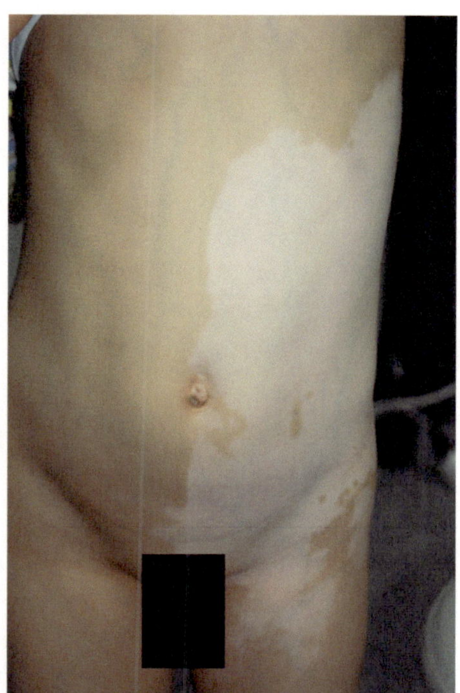

Fig. 6. Unilateral segmental vitiligo

of cases, and can affect the scalp, eyebrows and lashes, groin, and axillae (Hann & Lee, 1996; Hann, *et al.*, 1997). Extensive SV is very rare, and presents with involvement of over 50% of the body surface area (BSA) of the extremities and torso with facial sparing that is most often seen in early onset disease (van Geel, *et al.*, 2011). Autoimmune disease and atopy may or may not be associated with SV, unlike NSV.

3.2.1 Facial segmental vitiligo

As the face is the most common site for SV and the area causing the most psychological impact, it is important to know the exact spreading pattern and prognosis. Representatively, two classifications of facial SV have been proposed in order to suggest etiology of the SV and predict extent and location of involvement. The Hann classification is based on clinical patterns and their similarities, although some facial SV cannot be classified by this system. The Gauthier classification is based on the trigeminal dermatome.

Hann Classification

Hann *et al* classified facial SV into five types (Figure 7). *Type I* presents as subtype *A* or *B*, involvement begins on one side of the forehead, crosses the midline, and has downward spread over the opposite side of the face. *Type IA* occurs in 28.8% of facial vitiligo cases and primarily involves the mid-face with a predilection for the left side, although disease commonly crosses the midline. *Type IB* occurs in 10.5% of cases and involves the forehead, as well as frontal scalp and corresponding hair. Vitiligo is limited to above the eyebrows.

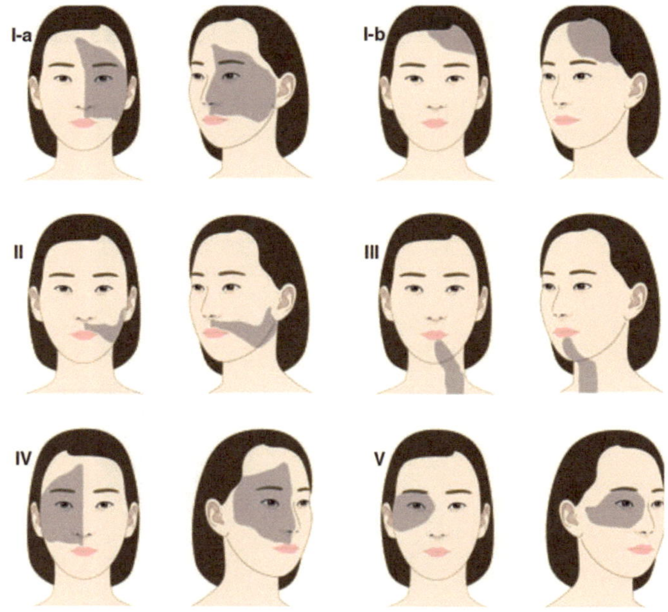

Fig. 7. Hann facial vitiligo classification. Adapted from *Hann SK, Kim DY, Oh SH. Classification of segmental vitiligo on the face: clues for prognosis. Brit J Dermatol 2011;164:1004-9.*

Type II has been reported in 16% of cases and originates in the infranasal area and spreads to the preauricular region. *Type III* is in 14.4% of cases and begins in the infralabial area and progresses towards the chin and neck. Nearly 11% of facial vitiligo is *Type IV*, which originates at the right forehead and involves the orbital, nasal, and buccal areas without crossing the midline. *Type V* is involvement of only the right orbital region, and occurs in 8.6% of cases (Hann, *et al.*, 2000; Hann, *et al.*, 2011).

Gauthier Classification

Gauthier developed another classification for face and neck SV (Figure 8). This is based on the trigeminal nerve distribution and involvement can be either partial or total: *Type I* (V1) corresponds to the ophthalmic region, *Type II* (V2) involves the maxillary area, and *Type III* (V3) refers to mandibular distribution. However, these types account for only 26% of cases, and the remaining majority involve overlapping areas of two or three dermatomes. *Type IV* (V1, V2, and V3) is subdivided into *4a*, involving V1 and V2, *4b*, involving V2 and V3, and *4c*, which involves the entire trigeminal dermatome. *Type V* refers to cases with the trigeminal nerve cervicofacial distribution (Gauthier Y, 2006).

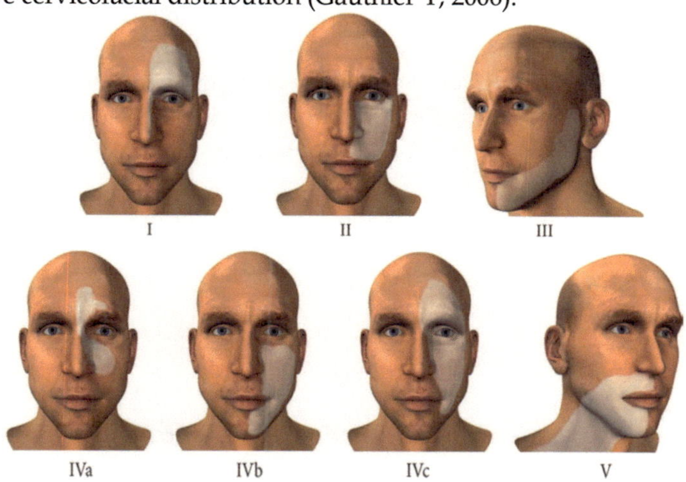

Fig. 8. Gauthier classification of segmental vitiligo of the face and neck. Adapted from *Hann SK, Gauthier Y, and Benzekri L. Segmental Vitiligo. In: Taïeb A, Picardo M, eds. Vitiligo. Berlin: Springer-Verlag Berlin Heidelberg: 2010.*

3.3 Mixed vitiligo

MV was initially presented by Hann and was proposed as a vitiligo classification by Taïeb and Picardo (Lee SJ, 2007). Spritz does not purport this classification, as MV presentation may represent the rare concurrence of NSV and SV which may be explained by shared genetic factors between NSV and SV.

MV is proposed as a classification because it is thought to be the progression of SV to a generalized form. This presentation may be due to an initial gene dysfunction that causes SV, which later triggers a general immune response in response to another genetic defect. The characteristics of MV are based on the observations of Taïeb and Picardo. They report that MV consists of SV involving at least 20% of its expected dermatome or in an obvious Blaschkolinear pattern, followed by the appearance of NSV at least 6 months later. The SV is more severe than the NSV while the generalized portion is generally mild (van Geel, *et al.*, 2011). The progression of SV to NSV can have varying periods of delay until presentation. In addition, compared to isolated SV, the SV portion of MV has limited face and neck involvement, with the thoraco-abdominal region as the most common location of disease (Hann & Lee, 1996; Ezzedine, *et al.*, 2011). There is no significant association with halo nevi and autoimmune disorders, although autoimmune disease is more common in MV than in pure SV (Taïeb & Picardo, 2007; Taïeb , *et al.*, 2008; van Geel, *et al.*, 2011). Furthermore, MV patients do not have a history of SV lesions at birth through 12 months of age, and the diagnosis of nevus depigmentosus has been excluded. Both pure SV and the SV of MV will typically respond poorly to narrowband ultraviolet B (NB-UVB) therapy while the NSV portions will respond well; this may reveal MV when the lesions of SV become apparent after NB-UVB treatment for NSV.

3.4 Mucosal vitiligo

Mucosal vitiligo can present as pure mucosal vitiligo, concurrently with NSV, or as part of acrofacial vitiligo. It is found in up to 50% of vitiligo patients with more pigmented skin types (Coondoo, *et al.*, 1976; Ortonne JP, 2002). Most commonly, mucosal vitiligo is on both lips, and in decreasing order of frequency, the isolated lower lip, glans penis, prepuce, angles of the mouth, labia minora, and hard palate and gums (Parsad, 2010). Other mucous membranes that can be involved are the oral mucosa, glans penis, prepuce, vulva, and anal mucosa. Disease is often resistant as the mucosal surfaces are non-hair-bearing and lack a melanocyte reservoir.

Pure mucosal vitiligo may represent a distinct type of vitiligo; it is observed to have a significantly older age of onset than patients with both cutaneous and mucosal involvement. It is also more common in smokers, which may reflect koebnerization due to mild thermal insult (Kanwar, *et al.*, 2010).

4. Halo nevi

The halo nevus is characterized by an amelanotic uniform ring around an acquired junctional, dermal, or compound nevus that is found in 1% of the general population. It seems to occur in similar rates in both NSV and SV (Barona, *et al.*, 1995). If halo nevi are concurrent with vitiligo, patients will report an earlier age of vitiligo onset and have less risk of autoimmune disease than those with isolated vitiligo (Taïeb & Picardo, 2007; Parsad, 2010). In addition, the associations with the Koebner phenomenon and the precipitating factors in common vitiligo associated with halo nevi are less than vitiligo without halo nevi. Furthermore, vitiligo associated with halo nevi did not show any positive associations with HLA-DR4 and DR53, which is a significant correlation (Taïeb & Picardo, 2007).

Individuals with three or more halo nevi for over 3 years, no personal or family history of vitiligo or autoimmune disease, and no evidence of koebnerization are at decreased risk for vitiligo (van Geel, *et al.*, 2011).

5. Leukotrichia, poliosis, and canities

Leukotrichia, or poliosis, is a focal patch of white hair that can occur in the background of chronic long-term vitiligo. It is commonly associated with rapidly progressive SV but is not a predictor of vitiligo prognosis (Hann, *et al.*, 1997).

Scalp poliosis is the most common presentation of hair involvement in vitiligo, followed by leukotrichia of the eyebrows, pubic hair, and axillae (Song MS, 1994).

Canities, or hair greying, has been associated with vitiligo. Early onset canities, occurring in individuals less than 30 years of age, may represent a form of vitiligo. Up to 37% of patients with vitiligo report premature canities. (Moscher DB, 1993; Ortonne JP, 2002)

6. Differential diagnosis

Vitiligo can be mistaken for a number of pigmentary disorders and dermatoses. A thorough history and physical examination is needed, and medical work-up should be a consideration. Vitiligo must be distinguished from genetic syndromes or disorders, nevus depigmentosus, idiopathic guttate hypomelanosis, piebaldism, infection-related hypomelanosis, progressive macular hypomelanosis, leukoderma (chemical, traumatic, or scleroderma), postinflammatory hypopigmentation, para-malignant hypomelanosis (*i.e.*, mycosis fungoides, melanoma), the effect of potent topical corticosteroid and drug-induced or occupational hypomelanosis, among others (Ortonne JP 2008).

7. Associated disorders and evaluation

Autoimmune and thyroid diseases are commonly associated with vitiligo, particularly in Caucasians (Silverberg, 2010). Almost one-third of vitiligo patients have a family member with autoimmune disease (Mason & Gawkrodger, 2005). Thyroid disease is most common, in particular hyper- (Grave's disease) or hypothyroidism (Hashimoto's thyroiditis). Other associations include alopecia areata, lichen sclerosis, Addison's disease, systemic lupus erythematous, rheumatoid arthritis, psoriasis, pernicious anemia, diabetes mellitus type II, gonadal failure, and inflammatory bowel disease (Ortonne JP, 2008; Achauer, 2003; Alkhateeb, *et al.*, 2003; Laberge, *et al.*, 2005). The genetic syndrome autoimmune polyendocrinopathy syndrome 1 (APS1), or autoimmune poly-endocrinopathy-candiasis ectodermal dystrophy (APECED), as well as the Vogt-Koyanagi-Harada (VKH) syndrome also feature vitiligo (Ortonne JP, 2008).

Patients with melanoma, both the cutaneous and ocular forms, can develop vitiligo, which is a positive prognostic indicator (Nordlund, *et al.*, 1983). Furthermore, ocular involvement manifesting as uveitis is not uncommon with vitiligo. Almost 20% of patients with concurrent vitiligo and melanoma have uveitis (Wagoner, *et al.*, 1983).

When a patient with vitiligo presents, it is apt exhaust the differential diagnosis as above in order to make an accurate clinical diagnosis. Due to the likelihood of potentially serious comorbidities, a medical work-up may be indicated (Table 2).

Test	Etiology	Frequency	Notes
Complete Blood Count	Macrocytic Anemia	Yearly	
Antinuclear antibody (ANA)	Autoimmune disease	Disease onset, low 25-hydroxy-vitamin D <15 ng/ml	Check prior to phototherapy initiation to rule out photosensitizing diseases
Chemistry panel	Diabetes mellitus, Addison's disease	Yearly	
25-Hydroxy-Vitamin D level	<15 ng/ml suggests work-up for autoimmune disease	Disease onset	Possible marker of secondary risk of autoimmune disease in vitiligo

Test	Etiology	Frequency	Notes
Homocysteine level	Elevated homocysteine level	As needed	Indicated for Middle Eastern, South American, Indian patients; vegetarian and other restricted diets
Thyroid stimulating hormone, free thyroxine, antithyroid peroxidase antibodies, antithyroglobulin antibodies	Thyroid disease	Yearly, positive patient or family history, symptomatic disease	Hypothyroidism most commonly associated with vitiligo
Folic acid	Folic acid deficiency	As needed	Indicated for alcoholics, low carbohydrate diets
Vitamin B6	Vitamin B6 deficiency	Elevated homocysteine level, rapid disease progression, photosensitivity with negative ANA	Check for history of medication use that interacts with Vitamin B6 (e.g., isoniazid)
Vitamin B12	Vitamin B12 deficiency	Elevated homocysteine levels, rapid disease progression, vegetarian diets	
Fasting blood sugar, insulin	Diabetes mellitus	High glucose levels, low 25-hydroxy-vitamin D level	

ng, nanogram

Table 2. Vitiligo Laboratory Evaluation

8. Special populations

8.1 Ethnic skin and skin of color

Vitiligo patches are more apparent on ethnic skin types (*i.e.*, Asian, black, and Hispanic) and skin of color, particularly Fitzpatrick skin types IV-VI (Halder & Chappell, 2009). These can cause much cosmetic concern and psychological distress due to the enhanced contrast of vitiligo on skin of color (Halder, *et al.*, 2003). This leads to stigmatization and the disease can be perceived as a threat to racial identity. Cultural values can also dictate the manner in which patients react to their disease. This may be the motivating factor for seeking treatment, and a culturally competent approach to these patients is warranted.

8.2 Pediatric vitiligo

It is estimated that more than half of vitiligo cases occur between the ages of 8-12 years old (Al-Mutairi, Sharma et al. 2005; Al-Mutairi, *et al.*, 2005) Nearly a third of children report a family history of vitiligo (Al-Mutairi, *et al.*, 2005). The most common type of vitiligo in pediatric cases is NSV, although children also have higher rates of SV than adults. The high rates of autoantibodies may be a predictor of autoimmune disease (Ortonne JP, 2008). NSV lesions are also sometimes accompanied by a hyperpigmented ring circumscribing lesions. Childhood SV is associated with a higher lesion count and involvement of a greater body surface area. There is no statistically significant difference in the frequency of reported triggering factors or poliosis between SV and NSV in children (Mazereeuw-Hautier, *et al.*, 2010).
Children are also greatly stigmatized by their disease, and during these formative years, it is of upmost concern that psychosocial issues be addressed. Adolescents, in particular, are more affected by their parents' perception of their vitiligo than by disease severity (Choi, *et al.*, 2010). Medical management of children differs from that of adults. It is recommended that therapy is rotated every 6-8 months with the addition of phototherapy as needed (Silverberg, 2010). Patient interactions should focus on providing encouragement and setting realistic treatment goals. A multidisciplinary approach to care, including other pediatric specialists (*e.g.*, endocrinologists, psychiatrists) is recommended for comprehensive care of these patients.

9. Psychosocial aspects & quality of life

The impact of vitiligo on each affected patient varies, but the disease is generally associated with significant psychological distress, disability, low self-esteem, and social isolation (Mattoo, *et al.*, 2002; Firooz, *et al.*, 2004). It can impair the health-related, sexual, and marital quality of life of patients (Papadopoulos, *et al.*, 1999; Firooz, *et al.*, 2004; Ongenae, *et al.*, 2005). A third of vitiligo patients have a psychiatric comorbidity, of which adjustment disorders and depression are most common (Porter, *et al.*, 1987; Agarwal, 1998; Mattoo, *et al.*, 2002). Women, patients with ethnic skin types or skin of color, and individuals with involvement in visible areas are prone to more severe psychological distress (Halder & Chappell, 2009).
Assessments of quality of life and the psychosocial effects of vitiligo on patients should be performed. Clinicians can be a source of support, and referral may be indicated. Psychological interventions including individual or group therapy, counseling (particularly for parents of children with vitiligo), cognitive behavioral therapy, and developing coping strategies with the patient can be useful (Thompson, *et al.*, 2002; Gawkrodger, *et al.*, 2010).

10. Conclusion

Vitiligo is a common amelanotic disorder that varies in presentation and can be associated with multiple medical conditions. A working knowledge of the characteristics of vitiligo, including its ability to impair quality of life, can guide management.

11. References

Achauer BM (2003). Carbon dioxide laser resurfacing and thin skin grafting in the treatment of stable and recalcitrant vitiligo. *Plast Reconstr Surg* 112: 1176.
Agarwal G (1998). Vitiligo: an under-estimated problem. *Fam Pract* 15 Suppl 1: S19-23.

Albert DM, Wagoner MD, Pruett RC, Nordlund JJ & Lerner AB (1983). Vitiligo and disorders of the retinal pigment epithelium. *Br J Ophthalmol* 67: 153-156.

Al-Mutairi N, Sharma AK, Al-Sheltawy M & Nour-Eldin O (2005). Childhood vitiligo: a prospective hospital-based study. *Australas J Dermatol* 46: 150-153.

Alkhateeb A, Fain PR, Thody A, Bennett DC & Spritz RA (2003). Epidemiology of vitiligo and associated autoimmune diseases in Caucasian probands and their families. *Pigment Cell Res* 16: 208-214.

Bang JS, Lee JW, Kim TH *et al.* (2000). Comparative clinical study of segmental and non segmental vitiligo. Kor J Dermatol 38:1037–1044.

Barona MI, Arrunategui A, Falabella R & Alzate A (1995). An epidemiologic case-control study in a population with vitiligo. *J Am Acad Dermatol* 33: 621-625.

Choi S, Kim DY, Whang SH, Lee JH, Hann SK & Shin YJ (2010). Quality of life and psychological adaptation of Korean adolescents with vitiligo. *J Eur Acad Dermatol Venereol* 24: 524-529.

Coondoo A, Sen N & Panja RK (1976). Leucoderma of the lips. A clinical study. *Indian J Dermatol* 21: 29-33.

el-Mofty AM & el-Mofty M (1980). Vitiligo. A symptom complex. *Int J Dermatol* 19: 237-244.

Esposito-Smythers C, Goldstein T, Birmaher B, *et al.* (2010) Clinical and psychosocial correlates of non-suicidal self-injury within a sample of children and adolescents with bipolar disorder. *J Affect Disord* 125: 89-97.

Moscher DB (1993). Vitiligo: etiology, pathogenesis, diagnosis and treatment. *Dermatology in general medicine,* Vol. 1 (Fitzpatrick TB EA, Wolff K, Freedberg AM, Austen KF, eds.), pp. McGraw Hill, New York.

Ezzedine K, Diallo A, Leaute-Labreze C, *et al.* (2011). Multivariate analysis of factors associated with early-onset segmental and nonsegmental vitiligo: a prospective observational study of 213 patients. *Br J Dermatol.*

Ezzedine K, Gauthier Y, Leaute-Labreze C, Marquez S, Bouchtnei S, Jouary T & Taïeb A (2011). Segmental vitiligo associated with generalized vitiligo (mixed vitiligo): A retrospective case series of 19 patients. *J Am Acad Dermatol.*

Firooz A, Bouzari N, Fallah N, Ghazisaidi B, Firoozabadi MR & Dowlati Y (2004). What patients with vitiligo believe about their condition. *Int J Dermatol* 43: 811-814.

Gauthier Y & Taïeb A (2006). Proposal for a new classification of segmental vitiligo of the face. *Pigment Cell Res* 19:515 (abstract).

Gauthier Y, Cario Andre M & Taïeb A (2003). A critical appraisal of vitiligo etiologic theories. Is melanocyte loss a melanocytorrhagy? *Pigment Cell Res* 16: 322-332.

Gawkrodger DJ, Ormerod AD, Shaw L, *et al.* (2010). Vitiligo: concise evidence based guidelines on diagnosis and management. *Postgrad Med J* 86: 466-471.

Halder RM (1997). Childhood vitiligo. *Clin Dermatol* 15: 899-906.

Halder RM & Chappell JL (2009). Vitiligo update. *Semin Cutan Med Surg* 28: 86-92.

Halder RM, Nandedkar MA & Neal KW (2003). Pigmentary disorders in ethnic skin. *Dermatol Clin* 21: 617-628, vii.

Hann SK, Kim DY & Oh SH (2011). Classification of segmental vitiligo on the face: clues for prognosis. *British Journal of Dermatology* 164: 1004-1009.

Hann SK, Chang JH, Lee HS & Kim SM (2000). The classification of segmental vitiligo on the face. *Yonsei Medical Journal* 41: 209-212.

Hann SK, Kim YS, Yoo JH & Chun YS (2000). Clinical and histopathologic characteristics of trichrome vitiligo. *J Am Acad Dermatol* 42: 589-596.

Hann SK, Chun WH & Park YK (1997). Clinical characteristics of progressive vitiligo. *Int J Dermatol* 36: 353-355.

Hann SK, Park YK & Chun WH (1997). Clinical features of vitiligo. *Clin Dermatol* 15: 891-897.

Hann SK & Lee HJ (1996) Segmental vitiligo: clinical findings in 208 patients. *J Am Acad Dermatol* 35: 671-674.

Ivker R, Goldaber M & Buchness MR (1994). Blue vitiligo. *J Am Acad Dermatol* 30: 829-831.

Karelson M, Silm H, Salum T, Koks S & Kingo K (2011). Differences between familial and sporadic cases of vitiligo. *J Eur Acad Dermatol Venereol.*

Kanwar A, Parsad D & De D (2010). Mucosal involvement in vitiligo: a comprehensive review of 241 cases. *J Eur Acad Dermatol Venereol.*

Koga M (1977). Vitiligo: a new classification and therapy. *Br J Dermatol* 97: 255-261.

Koga M & Tango T (1988). Clinical features and course of type A and type B vitiligo. *Br J Dermatol* 118: 223-228.

Kumarasinghe P. (2010). Vitiligo universalis. In Vitiligo, ed. Mauro Picardo and Alain Taïeb, 51-56. Berlin: Springer-Verlag Berlin Heidelberg.

Laberge G, Mailloux CM, Gowan K, Holland P, Bennett DC, Fain PR & Spritz RA (2005). Early disease onset and increased risk of other autoimmune diseases in familial generalized vitiligo. *Pigment Cell Res* 18: 300-305.

Lee SJ, Cho SB & Hann SK. (2007). Classification of vitiligo. In Surgical Management of Vitiligo, ed. Somesh Gupta, Mats J Olsson, Amrinder Kanwar, Jean-Paul Ortonne, 20-30. Oxford: Blackwell Publishing Ltd.

Lerner AB (1959). Vitiligo. *J Invest Dermatol* 32: 285-310.

Liu JB, Li M, Yang S, *et al.* (2005). Clinical profiles of vitiligo in China: an analysis of 3742 patients. *Clin Exp Dermatol* 30: 327-331.

Mason CP & Gawkrodger DJ (2005). Vitiligo presentation in adults. *Clin Exp Dermatol* 30: 344-345.

Mattoo SK, Handa S, Kaur I, Gupta N & Malhotra R (2002). Psychiatric morbidity in vitiligo: prevalence and correlates in India. *J Eur Acad Dermatol Venereol* 16: 573-578.

Mazereeuw-Hautier J, Bezio S, Mahe E, *et al.* (2010). Segmental and nonsegmental childhood vitiligo has distinct clinical characteristics: A prospective observational study. *Journal of the American Academy of Dermatology* 62: 945-949.

Nordlund JJ, Kirkwood JM, Forget BM, Milton G, Albert DM & Lerner AB (1983). Vitiligo in patients with metastatic melanoma: a good prognostic sign. *J Am Acad Dermatol* 9: 689-696.

Ongenae K, Dierckxsens L, Brochez L, van Geel N & Naeyaert JM (2005). Quality of life and stigmatization profile in a cohort of vitiligo patients and effect of the use of camouflage. *Dermatology* 210: 279-285.

Ortonne JP. (2002). Depigmentation of hair and mucous membrane. In Vitiligo, ed. Seung-Kyung Hann and James J. Nordlund, 76-80. Oxford: Blackwell Science.

Ortonne JP. (2008). Vitiligo and other disorders of hypopigmentation. In: Dermatology, ed. Jean L. Bolognia, Joseph L. Jorizzo, Ronald P. Rapini, 913-938. New York, NY: Mosby.

Papadopoulos L, Bor R & Legg C (1999). Coping with the disfiguring effects of vitiligo: a preliminary investigation into the effects of cognitive-behavioural therapy. *Br J Med Psychol* 72 (Pt 3): 385-396.

Park K, Youn JL, Lee YS (1988). A clinical study of 326 cases of vitiligo. *Korean J Dermatol* 26:200–205.

Parsad D. (2010). Mucosal vitiligo. In Vitiligo, ed. Mauro Picardo and Alain Taïeb, 57-59. Berlin: Springer-Verlag Berlin Heidelberg.

Passeron T & Ortonne JP. (2010). Generalized vitiligo. In Vitiligo, ed. Mauro Picardo and Alain Taïeb, 35-39. Berlin: Springer-Verlag Berlin Heidelberg.

Porter J, Beuf AH, Lerner A & Nordlund J (1987). Response to cosmetic disfigurement: patients with vitiligo. *Cutis* 39: 493-494.

Silverberg NB (2010). Update on childhood vitiligo. *Curr Opin Pediatr* 22: 445-452.

Silverberg NB & Travis L (2006). Childhood vitiligo. *Cutis* 77: 370-375.

Song MS HS, Ahn PS *et al.* (1994). Clinical study of vitiligo: comparative study of type A and type B vitiligo. Ann Dermatol (Seoul) 6:22–30.

Taïeb A & Picardo M (2010). Epidemiology, definitions, classification. *Vitiligo,*(Taïeb A PM, eds.), pp. Springer-Verlag Berlin Heidelberg, Berlin

Taïeb A & Picardo M (2009). Clinical practice. Vitiligo. *N Engl J Med* 360: 160-169.

Taïeb A & Picardo M (2007). The definition and assessment of vitiligo: a consensus report of the Vitiligo European Task Force. *Pigment Cell Res* 20: 27-35.

Taïeb A, Morice-Picard F, Jouary T, Ezzedine K, Cario-Andre M & Gauthier Y (2008). Segmental vitiligo as the possible expression of cutaneous somatic mosaicism: implications for common non-segmental vitiligo. *Pigment Cell Melanoma Res* 21: 646-652.

Thompson AR, Kent G & Smith JA (2002). Living with vitiligo: dealing with difference. *Br J Health Psychol* 7: 213-225.

van Geel N, De Lille S, Vandenhaute S, Gauthier Y, Mollet I, Brochez L & Lambert J (2011). Different phenotypes of segmental vitiligo based on a clinical observational study. *J Eur Acad Dermatol Venereol* 25: 673-678.

van Geel N, Vandenhaute S, Speeckaert R, Brochez L, Mollet I, De Cooman L & Lambert J (2011). Prognostic value and clinical significance of halo naevi regarding vitiligo. *Br J Dermatol* 164: 743-749.

Wagoner MD, Albert DM, Lerner AB, Kirkwood J, Forget BM & Nordlund JJ (1983). New observations on vitiligo and ocular disease. *Am J Ophthalmol* 96: 16-26.

1

Genetic Epidemiology and Heritability of Vitiligo

Abdullateef A. Alzolibani[1], Ahmad Al Robaee[1] and Khaled Zedan[2]
[1]*Department Of Dermatology, College Of Medicine, Qassim University*
[2]*Pediatric Department, College Of Medicine, Qassim University*
Saudi Arabia

1. Introduction

1.1 Prevalence & incidence

The population prevalence of vitiligo ranges from 0.1% to 2% and shows a wide variability among ethnic groups (Bolognia et al., 1998; Hann and Nordlund, 2000). Whereas the estimated population prevalence of vitiligo is approximately 0.38% for Caucasians in the United States and Northern Europe (Howitz et al., 1977), vitiligo affects 0.19% of the population in China (Xu et al., 2002). Other international studies show that the incidence of vitiligo ranges from 0.1 to over 8.8% (Srivastava, 1994; Schwartz and Janniger, 1997; Hann et al., 1997; Kovacs, 1998; Agarwal, 1998; Handa and Kaur, 1999; Alkhateeb et al., 2003). The highest incidence of the condition has been recorded in Indians from the Indian subcontinent, followed by Mexico and Japan (Table 1). The difference in its incidence may be due to higher reporting of vitiligo in a population, where an apparent color contrast and stigma attached to the condition may force patients to seek early consultation (Panja, 1947; Levai, 1958; Punshi and Thakre, 1969; Behl and Bhatia, 1971; Sehgal, 1974; Koranne and Sachdeva, 1988; El Mofty, 1968; Grunnet et al., 1970; Dawber, 1968; Perrot, 1973; Fornara, 1941; Canizares, 1960; Ruiz Maldonnado et al., 1977; Fitzpatrick, 1974; Arakawa, 1941; Khoo, 1962).

Vitiligo is reported more frequently in females than males, which may be the result of increased reporting rates in females due to greater social consequences in females affected by vitiligo (Kovacs, 1998; Lee Poole and Boissy, 1997; Hann and Lee, 1996; Zaima and Koga, 2002; Jeninger, 1993; Halder, 1997; Cho et al., 2000; Handa and Dogra, 2003).

Adults and children of both sexes are equally affected; however, the majority of the vitiligo cases are reported during stages of active development. About 50% of patients present before the age of 20 and nearly 70-80% present before 30 years of age. Although no age is immune to vitiligo, the disease is very rarely observed at birth (Behl et al., 2003; Jaigirdar et al., 2002; Engel, 2001; Lerner, 1999; Gauthier et al., 2003; Westerhof et al., 1996).

The proportion of patients with a positive family history varies from one part of the world to another, with particularly wide ranges reported in India (6.25-18%), with reports of up to 40% elsewhere in the world (Behl et al., 2003).

Author(s)	Year	City/ or Region/Country/Continent	Incidence (%)
El Mofty	1968	Egypt/Africa	1
Panja	1947	Calcutta/India/Asia	6
Levai	1958	Vellore/India/Asia	4
Punshi & Thakre	1969	Amrawati/India/Asia	8
Behl & Bhatia	1972	Delhi/India/Asia	8.8
Sehgal	1974	Goa/India/Asia	2.9
Koranne &Sachdeva	1988	Delhi/India/Asia`	1.25
Howitz *et al.*	1977	Denmark/Europe	0.38
Grunnet *et al.*	1970	Denmark/Europe	1.44
Dawber	1968	England/Europe	0.15
Perrot	1973	France/Europe	3.0
Fornara	1941	Italy/Europe	0.3
Canizares	1960	Mexico/North America	4
Ruiz-Maldonnado	1977	Mexico/North America	2.6
Fitzpatrick	1974	Massachusetts/United States/North America	8
Arakawa	1941	Japan/Asia	1.64
Khoo	1962	Malaysia/Asia	0.7

Table 1. Vitiligo: Global Incidence Patterns

2. Epidemiology of vitiligo: A worldwide survey

Numerous studies have been conducted around the world concerning the epidemiological characteristics of vitiligo, in particular the racial, ethnic, and cultural differences in its prevalence.

2.1 Europe

2.1.1 Denmark

The prevalence of vitiligo was 0.38% in a representative population of 47,033 in Denmark. Both sexes were found to be equally affected, with no significant difference found in the distribution of vitiligo patients among five different municipalities or between urban and rural districts. New cases of vitiligo steadily increased with advancing age, its onset being most often between the ages of 40 and 60 years of age. The age-specific prevalence increased from 0.09% in patients under the age of 10 to 0.9% in the age group between 60 to 69 years. It was suggested that these characteristics of vitiligo in Denmark would also apply to northwest Europe (Howitz et al., 1977).

2.1.2 United Kingdom

The characteristics of vitiligo in 41 adults presenting to a university dermatology clinic in Sheffield, United Kingdom were studied in a case review. Of 41 patients, there were 29 women (70.7%) and 12 men (29.3). The authors reported an age of onset before 20 years in 41.5% of patients (n=17), while the mean was 28 years. The oldest age of onset was 74 years. In these patients, the average duration of disease was 16 years. Autoimmune thyroid disease was present in 34.1% of cases (n=14). Only 17% (n=7) gave a family history of vitiligo (Mason and Gawk Rodger, 2005).

2.2 Middle East

2.2.1 Saudi Arabia: Qassim region

Alzolibani found that in a random sampling of vitiligo patients in the Qassim region of Saudi Arabia, approximately one-third of cases were positive for parental consan`guinity.

A particularly high first-cousin consanguinity was noted in this study, which was found to be higher than that reported among the general Saudi population (22.5% vs. 19.5%) (Alzolibani, 2009; El-Hazmi et al., 1995).

Moreover, a positive family history was obtained in 56.8% of families studied, 57.1% of them having two or more affected relatives. The age of onset of vitiligo was 31 years in familial cases and 33 years in non-familial controls. Vitiligo occurred before the age of 20 in 19% of family cases and in 36% of non-familial controls. Most families (75%) had no more than two affected members.

As observed in this study, the incidence rate of vitiligo in relatives increased with a closer blood relationship to probands, which is indicative of the significant familial aggregation of vitiligo noted in a number of previous studies (Nath et al., 1994; Majumder et al., 1988). The proband cases in this study showed higher relative risks among their first- and second-degree relatives, but not as high among their third-degree relatives.

Inheritance pattern prediction using the frequency of vitiligo among siblings in relation to the general population coincided with the multifactorial model particularly for the vitiligo vulgaris subtype followed by the acrofacial subtype, and least in the focal subtype. Calculation of heritability showed a high weighted mean of 0.54.

Similar data from China supports these findings (Sun et al., 2006).

Genetic factors play a relatively important role in the evolution of vitiligo among subjects in the Qassim region. Recognition of this could have a potential impact on disease prevention through family counseling and other forms of intervention.

2.2.2 Kuwait

In a sample of 88 pediatric vitiligo patients at a hospital dermatology clinic, the age of onset was between 8 and 12 years in 51% of these patients (Al-Mutairi et al., 2005). A positive family history was obtained in 27.3% of the patients. Vitiligo vulgaris was the most common clinical type observed. Three patients, though clinically asymptomatic, incidentally had anti-thyroid antibodies, which are comparable to results published previously.

Eighty Korean children (ages 8 months-12 years) with clinical and/or histopathologic diagnoses of vitiligo were evaluated; :39 boys and 41 girls. The mean age at first visit was 7.9 years and the mean age at disease onset was 5.6 years. The children were compared with a control group of 422 adults with vitiligo. Children comprised 16% of the total vitiligo patients and adults comprised 84%. A family history of vitiligo was found in 11 (13.8%) of children, compared to 10.7% in the adult group. ; pPoliosis was found in 20 (25%) of children. H; halo nevi was found in 2 (2.5%) of children, compared to 4% in the adult group; combined autoimmune and endocrine diseases were noted in in 1 (1.3% of children), compared to 7.6% in the adult group; and segmental vitiligo in 26 (was diagnosed in 32.5% of children), compared to 13.0% inof the adult group. TheVitiligo and its associated conditions were combined diseases were significantly less often frequentfound in children compared tothan adults ($p < 0.01$), and segmental vitiligo was found in significantly higher numbers of children than the adult patientsmore often associated with children ($p < 0.0001$). Thise study does id not show a higher prevalence of vitiligo in girls as reported in other studies, which may indicate a racial differencetrait (Cho et al., 2000).

2.3 Indian subcontinent

2.3.1 India

In India, the incidence of vitiligo was reported to be between 1- 2 % (Majumder et al., 1988). In a large population-based study of vitiligo patients (n=998), 43% were male (n=429) and (57%) were females (n=569). The mean age at onset for males was found to be 23.3 years and for females was 17.4 years. The median age at onset in males was 18 years and 13.6 years in females. The earliest age at onset was found to be at birth and the oldest was 73 years (Tawade et al., 1997).Out of 998 cases, 272 (27.3%) had one or more relatives with vitiligo. Among these, 207 (76.1%) cases had only one relative affected whereas 65 (28%) cases had more than one relative with vitiligo.

The slightly higher prevalence in females may not be the true situation, as only self-reported cases were enlisted in the study. Due to the social stigma of vitiligo in the community, young females tend to report earlier due to matrimonial anxiety. The age at onset is consistent with previous studies (Mosher et al., 1987). Onset at birth is not so common. In the present study 3 cases had onset of vitiligo at birth, of which One infant's mother had vitiligo. The peak incidence between 5-14 years may reflect concerns about cosmetic disfigurement in this age group and parental anxiety leading to early reporting.

In another Indian study (Handa and Kaur, 1999), 1,436 patients were seen between 1989 and 1993. Males constituted 54.5% of the group and females, 45.5%. Mean age of the patients was 25 years, and average disease duration at the time of hospital visit was 3.7 years. Leukotrichia was present in 165 (11.5%), and Koebner's phenomenon was observed in 72 (5.0%). Twenty-nine (2%) patients had associated halo nevi. A family history of vitiligo was reported in 165 (11.5%) patients.

A study was performed in a military service hospital patient population utilizing 120 cases of vitiligo (Kar, 2001). The youngest patient in this series was a 2 year-old girl and oldest patient was 65 year old male. In 52 (43.2%) patients, disease started before the age of 20. The duration of disease varied from 2 months to ten years. Eight patients (6.6%) reported a family history of vitiligo. In one case, a mother and her two daughters had vitiligo. The male -to -female ratio in vitiligo was observed in this study to be nearly equal, meaning thereby this disease had no predilection for any gender. Similar observations were also noted by various researchers (Sarin and Kumar, 1977; Behl et al., 1961). Furthermore, the incidence of vitiligo was 43.2% in the age group of 20 years of age and younger, as compared to an incidence of 9.9% in individuals over 40 years of age. Universal vitiligo was found in 2 (1.6%) cases and both had a positive family history of disease. Other studies found a positive family history in 6.25-10% of cases (Sarin and

Kumar, 1977; Behl et al., 1961). The results of this study may indicate that the mode of vitiligo transmission may be caused by an autosomal dominant gene with variable penetrance (Ando et al., 1993; Behl et al., 1994).

In an Indian pediatric population (Handa and Dogra, 2003), 625 children with vitiligo were seen over 10 years: 357 (57.1%) were girls and 268 (42.9%) were boys. As compared to adult patients with vitiligo, this sex difference was found to be statistically significant ($p < 0.001$). The mean age of onset of the disease was 6.2 years. Leukotrichia was present in 77 patients (12.3%), while Koebner phenomenon was observed in 71 patients (11.3%). Halo nevi were observed in 29 patients (4.4%). Seventy-six patients (12.2%) had a family history of vitiligo.

A total of 365 patients were included in a study that focused on the clinical and sociodemographic aspects of vitiligo. There was a female preponderance of disease: females (68.4%) were found to be more affected than males (31.6%), in a ratio of 2.1:1 (Shah et al., 2008). The majority (32.82%) of the patients were in their second decade of life, and 58.63% of the patients were unmarried. A positive family history was present in 50 (13.7%) of patients, and first-degree relatives were affected in 35 of these patients. Vitiligo has a polygenic or autosomal dominant inheritance pattern with incomplete penetrance and variable expression (Bleehen et al., 1992; Moscher et al., 1993; Bolognia and Pawelek, 1988). Familial occurrence has been reported to be in the range of 6.25% to 30% (Shajil et al., 2006). Positive family history is considered to be a poor prognostic factor for vitiligo.

The female-to-male ratio in this study was 2.1:1, which was different from other study findings (Handa and Kaur, 1999; Koranne et al., 1986). Most reports showed that males and females were affected with almost equal frequency, but females outnumbered males in this study presumably because of social stigma and the marital concerns which prompt women to seek early consultation. In 54.5% of the patients, the age at onset was in the first or second decade of life, consistent with most reports from India and the West.

2.3.2 Mumbai

In Mumbai, India, records of 33,252 new patients attending a dermatology outpatient department from June 2002 to June 2008 were analyzed for the presence of vitiligo (Poojary, 2011).

The total number of vitiligo patients was 204. The male: female proportion was almost equal. A family history of vitiligo was seen in 3.43% of cases. Associated autoimmune disorders were seen in 2.94% of cases and were mainly skin associated autoimmune diseases (morphea, alopecia areata, discoid lupus erythematosus, and pemphigus erythematosus), except for one case of Grave's disease. This may indicate that the association of vitiligo with other autoimmune diseases emphasizes the autoimmune etiology of vitiligo, and also the need to actively look for, and if necessary, investigate patients with vitiligo for other autoimmune diseases.

2.3.3 Calcutta

An epidemiological profile of vitiligo in Calcutta was gathered from 15,685 individuals drawn from the general population; pedigree data was collected from 293 vitiligo patients. The overall prevalence of vitiligo was about 5 per 1,000 individuals. There were no significant sex or age differences. About a 4.5-fold increase in prevalence was observed among close biological relatives of affected individuals. There were no significant differences in the frequencies of various types of vitiligo between probands with and without positive family history. The overall mean and modal ages of onset were about 22 years and 15 years, respectively. The mean ages among males (24.8 years) and females (19.3 years) were significantly different (Das et al., 1985).

2.4 Africa

2.4.1 Tunisia

In a retrospective study of patients attending a Tunisian outpatient dermatological practice (Zeglaoui et al., 1985), 503 patients were reviewed from a 5-year period. There were 288 women (57.3%) and 215 (42.7%) men (F: M = 1.33). The average age was 28.2 years (3- 80 years). The peak of frequency was located in the second decade of the life (26%). A family history of vitiligo was found in 27% of cases. The average time of until initial consultation was 21 months. An association with other pathological conditions was found in 23% of cases which is consistent with available literature.

2.4.2 Nigeria

To investigate vitiligo in the Nigerian Africans, 351 patients with vitiligo, representing 3.2% of new dermatologic cases at a study wsite, were enrolled (Onunu and Kubeyinje, 2003). The study group was made up of 153 males (43.6%) and 198 females (56.4), giving a sex ratio of 1: 1.3. The peak incidence of vitiligo was in the second and third decades of life. There was a positive family history of vitiligo in 18% of subjects.

2.5 Caribbean

2.5.1 French West Indies: Isle of Martinique

A study was conducted in an academic dermatology clinic which analyzed a cohort of 2,077 dermatology outpatients. There was a vitiligo prevalence rate of 0.34%, with a predominance of affected females. The median age at onset was 29 years. Of the vitiligo patients, over 30% had a family history of vitiligo, 6% (n=2) had concurrent thyroid disease, 6% (n=2) had psoriasis, and 3% (n=1) had atopic dermatitis. These findings are comparable to data in Caucasian populations (Boisseau-Garsaud et al., 2000).

2.6 North America

2.6.1 United States

Data on 160 Caucasian families living in the United States was collected based on primary probands with vitiligo (Majumder et al., 1993). The rate at which first degree relatives were also afflicted with vitiligo is 20%. Children of probands were found to have 1.7 times the risk of vitiligo compared to other first-degree relatives. The relative risk (RR) for vitiligo was approximately 7 for parents, 12 for siblings, and 36 for children. For second-degree relatives, the RR varied between 1 and 16. The pattern of the relationship between RR and degree of kinship indicates the involvement of genetic factors, although it is not consistent with single-locus Mendelian transmission.

In general, patients with vitiligo who have an family history of vitiligo are more likely to have an earlier age of onset of disease than those with a negative family history (odds ratio = 3.70, P = .024). There was found to be no association between family history and site of onset, distribution, or course of disease. Onset of pediatric vitiligo also seemed to be linked to a family history of vitiligo. This suggests that awareness of this association can allow for earlier detection and initiation of treatment (Pajvani et al., 2006)

3. Genetic heritability of vitiligo

3.1 Familial aggregation of vitiligo and relationship with autoimmune diseases

Familial aggregation of vitiligo was noted as early as 1933 (Majumder, 2000), suggesting that genetic factors might have an important effect on the development of vitiligo (Hafez et al., 1983). Although vitiligo aggregates in families, it does not appear to segregate in a simple Mendelian pattern (Majumder et al., 1993; Kim et al., 1997; Nordlund and Majumder, 1997). Previously, an autosomal recessive model of vitiligo that took the variability of the age of onset into account was proposed, suggesting that there might be genes at three or four autosomal loci controlling vitiligo (Alkhateeb et al., 2002; Majumder et al., 1988). This was supported by the high frequency of vitiligo and other autoimmune diseases in isolated inbred communities. On the other hand, the actual onset of vitiligo in genetically susceptible individuals seems to require exposure to environmental triggers (Nath et al., 1994; Birela et al., 2008). Attempts to identify genes involved in vitiligo susceptibility have involved gene expression studies, allelic association studies of candidate genes, and genome-wide linkage analyses to discover new genes (Zhang et al., 2008).

Most evidence indicates that generalized vitiligo is an organ-specific autoimmune disease directed against melanocytes (Ongenae et al., 2003; Rezaei et al., 2007), and indeed about 20% of vitiligo patients (and their close relatives) manifest concomitant occurrence of other autoimmune diseases, particularly autoimmune thyroid disease, rheumatoid arthritis, late-onset type I diabetes mellitus, psoriasis, pernicious anemia, systemic lupus erythematosus, and Addison's disease (Alkhateeb et al., 2003). Nevertheless, heritable biological properties of the melanocyte or other factors, combined with environmental triggers, may contribute to loss of immune tolerance and ultimately autoimmunity directed against melanocytes (Boissy and Spritz, 2009). Family clusters of vitiligo cases are not uncommon, occurring in a non-Mendelian pattern suggestive of polygenic, multifactorial inheritance. Probands' first-degree relatives have 6–7% risk of developing generalized vitiligo, and the concordance rate in monozygotic twins is 23%.

Genetic linkage and association studies have implicated a number of genes in vitiligo pathogenesis, especially genes involved in immune function (Spritz, 2007; Spritz, 2008). However, these loci account for a relatively small fraction of total disease liability. Genetically isolated "founder populations" afford special opportunities to identify genes involved in susceptibility to disease, as founder populations may have elevated prevalence of specific diseases and reduced heterogeneity of causal genetic and environmental risk factors compared with more outbred populations (Wright et al., 1999). Accordingly, susceptibility alleles that represent relatively minor genetic risk factors for complex diseases in the general population may become amplified and constitute major risk alleles in a founder population, and thus may be localized using less dense maps and smaller sample sizes than similar studies conducted in more outbred populations (Wittke-Thompson et al., 2007).

3.2 Genetic basis of vitiligo

Genes play a role in all aspects of vitiligo pathogenesis, even in response to environmental triggers. Typical generalized vitiligo behaves as a "complex trait", meaning it is a polygenic, multifactorial disease involving multiple genes and non-genetic factors. Only a few vitiligo susceptibility genes have been identified with reasonable certainty. These include human leukocyte antigen (HLA), protein tyrosine phosphatase, non-receptor type 22 (*PTPN22),* and, *NACHT, LRR and PYD domains-containing protein 1 (NALP1)*, all genes associated with autoimmune susceptibility. Cytotoxic lymphocyte antigen 4 (*CTLA4)* is also under investigation (Spitz, 2008).

The earliest evidence suggesting a genetic basis for vitiligo was its association with a number of other autoimmune disorders known to have heritable predispositions, such as type 1 diabetes mellitus. Furthermore, genetic diseases are substantially more prevalent in children of parents who are close relatives. In an Indian study of a community with a predominance of consanguineous marriages, 20% of individuals had vitiligo (Ramaiah et al., 1988). Significantly earlier onset has been observed when there is a family history of vitiligo (24.8 vs. 42.2 years of age) (Hann and Lee, 1996).

Genetic models suggested by analysis of family studies include a multifactorial model (Goudie et al., 1983), a dominant model with incomplete penetration (Hafez et al., 1983), and a multilocular recessive model (Majumder et al., 1988). There may also be two coexisting modes of inheritance for vitiligo depending on age of onset (Arcos-Burgos et al., 2002). In patients with early onset vitiligo (before the age of 30), vitiligo inheritance most closely follows a dominant mode of inheritance with incomplete penetration. However, a predisposition for vitiligo resulting from a recessive genotype and exposure to certain environmental triggers appears to explain the inheritance pattern of late onset vitiligo (after 30 years of age). Specific HLA haplotypes are strongly associated with family history of vitiligo, severity of disease, age of onset, and population geography (Zamani et al., 2001; Ando et al., 1993; Finco et al., 1991). Gene polymorphisms in the major histocompatibility complex (MHC) Class II region of the HLA locus have been previously found to be associated with other autoimmune diseases, such as type 1 diabetes mellitus and juvenile-onset rheumatoid arthritis (Deng et al., 1995; Prahalad et al., 2001). The HLA genes encoding both the transporter associated with antigen-processing (*TAP1*) and subunits of the immunoproteasome latent membrane protein 2 and 7 (*LMP2/LMP7*) have been found to be associated with vitiligo of early onset in Caucasian patients (Casp et al., 2003).

The (*CTLA-4*) gene encodes a protein involved in the inhibition of improperly-activated T-cells. *CTLA-4* variants have been linked to numerous autoimmune diseases. There is an association between the *CTLA-4* polymorphism and the occurrence of vitiligo with other autoimmune comorbidities (Blomhoff et al., 2005). Catechol-O-methyl transferase (*CTLA-4*) is an enzyme that plays a major role in the metabolism of toxic or biologically active drugs, neurotransmitters and metabolites. One such metabolite, O-quinones, can be formed during melanin synthesis in the absence of adequate *CTLA-4* activity. A *CTLA-4* polymorphism has been found to be significantly associated with acrofacial vitiligo (Tursen et al., 2002).

Chromosome 1p31, termed the autoimmune susceptibility locus (*AIS1*), has been found to be associated to a highly significant degree with generalized vitiligo in Caucasians living in North American and the United Kingdom (Fain et al., 2003). Reduced activity of the *VIT1* gene, located on chromosome 2p16, has been associated with increased susceptibility to vitiligo, possibly as a result of dysfunction of melanocyte nucleotide mismatch repair(Lee Poole, 2001).

A genome-wide association study of generalized vitiligo in an isolated European founder population identified a significant association of single-nucleotide polymorphisms in a block on band 6q27, in close vicinity to IDDM8, which is a linkage and an association signal for type I diabetes mellitus and rheumatoid arthritis. Only one gene, SMOC2, is in the region of association, within which single-nucleotide polymorphism (SNP) rs13208776 attained genome-wide significance for association with other autoimmune diseases and vitiligo (Birlea et al., 2009).

Genetic risk for vitiligo is well-supported by multiple lines of evidence. Vitiligo is frequently associated with familial clustering (Alkhateeb et al., 2003; Goudie et al., 1983; Mehta et al., 1973; Carnevale et al., 1980). Approximately 20% of probands have at least one affected first degree relative. The risk of first degree relatives of patients with vitiligo for developing the disease is elevated by 7- to 10-fold compared to the general population (Alkhateeb et al., 2003; Sun et al. 2006).

In addition, segregation analysis suggests that vitiligo is a multifactorial and polygenic disorder that likely results from multiple genetic and environmental factors (Alkhateeb et al., 2003; Arcos-Burgos et al., 2002; Nath et al., 2001; Spritz et al., 2004). However, no disease genes have been identified for vitiligo thus far. Several genome-wide linkage analyses of vitiligo have been performed in the past few years, and multiple linkages to vitiligo have been identified (Alkhateeb et al., 2002; Fain et al., 2003; Spritz et al., 2004). Co-segregation of systemic lupus erythematosus and vitiligo in European American pedigrees revealed significant linkage on 17p13 (Nath et al., 2001). Another co-segregation of vitiligo and Hashimoto thyroiditis identified a candidate gene with highly significant linkage at a locus ("*AIS1*") on chromosome 1p32.2-p31.3 (Alkhateeb et al., 2002; Spritz et al., 2004), as well as additional linkage evidence on chromosomes 1, 7, 8, 11, 19, and 22 (Spritz et al., 2004). There are confirmed linkage findings on chromosomes 7q and 8p (*AIS2 and AIS3*) (Nath et al., 2001). The linkage evidence at the *AIS1, AIS2,* and systemic lupus erythematosus, vitiligo-related 1 (*SLEV1)* loci was mainly from autoimmunity-associated families, while the evidence at the *AIS3* locus was primarily from non-autoimmunity-associated families, suggesting that generalized vitiligo may be divided into two distinct phenotypic subcategories that involve different disease loci or alleles.

4. Conclusion

Vitiligo is a common, acquired, discoloration of the skin. Most studies show that vitiligo is common in the younger age group, with females of reproductive age forming the major group. Genetic factors play a relatively important role in the evolution of vitiligo. The extent of familial aggregation of vitiligo is statistically significant. The genetic model of vitiligo may be consistent with a polygenetic or multifactorial inheritance in a dominant gene pattern.

5. References

Agarwal G. Vitiligo: An under-estimated problem. Fam Pract 1998;15:519-23.

Akay BN, Bozkir M, Anadolu Y, Gullu S. Epidemiology of vitiligo, associated autoimmune diseases and audiological abnormalities: Ankara study of 80 patients in Turkey. J Eur Acad Dermatol venereal. 2010 Oct;24(10):1144-50.

Alkhateeb A, Fain PR, Thody A, Bennett DC, Spritz RA. Epidemiology of vitiligo and associated autoimmune diseases in Caucasian probands and their families. Pigment Cell Res 2003;16:208-14.

Alkhateeb A, Stetler GL, Old W, Talbert J, Uhlhorn C, Taylor M, et al. Mapping of an autoimmunity susceptibility locus (AIS1) to chromosome 1p31.3–p32.2. Hum Mol Genet. 2002; 11:661–7.

Al-mutairi N, Sharma AK, Al-Sheltawy M, Nour-Eldin O. Childhood vitiligo: a prospective hospital-based study. Australas J. 2005 Aug;46(3):150-3.

Alzolibani A. Genetic epidemiology and heritability of vitiligo in the Qassim region of Saudi Arabia. Acta Dermatovenerol Alp Panonica Adriat. 2009 Sep;18(3):119-25.

Ando-I, Chi-HI, Nakagawa H, et al. Differences in clinical features and HLA antigens between familial and non familial vitiligo of non segmental type. Br J Dermatol 1993; 123:408-410.

Arakawa A. Quoted by Robert P. Uber die Vitiligo, Dermatologica 1941;84:257-319.

Arcos-Burgos M. Parodi E. Salgar M. Bedoya E. Builes J. Jaramillo D. Ceballos G. Uribe A. Rivera N. Rivera D. Fonseca I. Camargo M. Palacio G. Vitiligo: complex segregation and linkage disequilibrium analyses with respect to microsatellite loci spanning the HLA. Hum Genet 2002; 110: 334-42.

Arycan O, Koc K, Ersoy L. Clinical characteristics in 113 Turkish vitiligo patients. Acta dermatovenerol Alp Panonica Adriat. 2008 Sep; 17(3):129-32.

Behl PN, Agarwal RS, Singh G. Etiological studies in vitiligo and therapeutic response to standard treatment. Indian J Dermatol 1961;6:101.

Behl PN, Aggarwal A, Srivastava G. Vitiligo *In* : Behl PN, Srivastava G, editors. Practice of Dermatology. 9 th ed. CBS Publishers: New Delhi; 2003. p. 238-41.

Behl PN, Bhatia RK. 400 case of vitiligo - A clinico therapeutic analysis. Indian J Dermatol 1971;17:51-4.

Behl PN, Kotia A, Sawal P. Vitiligo: Age group related trigger factor and morphological variants. Indian J Dermatol Venereol Lepr 1994;60: 275-279.

Birlea SA, Fain PR, Spritz RA. A Romanian population isolate with high frequency of vitiligo and associated autoimmune diseases. Arch Dermatol. 2008 Mar;144(3):310–6.

Birlea SA, Gowan K, Fain PR, Spritz RA. Genome-Wide Association Study of Generalized Vitiligo in an Isolated European Founder Population Identifies SMOC2, in Close Proximity to IDDM8. *J Invest Dermatol*. Nov 5 2009.

Bleehen SS, Ebling FJ, Champion RH. Disorders of skin color. *In* : Champion RH, Burton JL, Ebling FJ, editors. Text book of Dermatology. London: Blackwell Scientific Publications; 1992. p. 1561-622.

Blomhoff A. Helen Kemp E. Gawkrodger DJ. Weetman AP. Husebye ES. Akselsen HE. Lie BA. Undlien DE. CTLA4 polymorphisms. Pigment Cell Res 2005; 18: 55-8.

Boisseau-Garsaud AM, Garsaud P, Cales-Quist D, Helenon R, Queneherve C, Clair RC. Epidemiology of vitiligo in the French West Indies (Isle of Martinique). Int J Dermatol. 2000 Jan;39(1):18-20.

Boissy RE, Spritz RA (2009) Frontiers and controversies in the pathobiology of vitiligo: separating the wheat from the chaff. Exp Dermatol 18:583–5

Bolognia JL, Nordlund JJ, Ortonne J-P (1998) Vitiligo vulgaris.In: Nordlund JJ, Boissy RE, Hearing VJ, King RA, Ortonne J-P (eds) The pigmentary system. Oxford UniversityPress, New York, pp 513–551.

Bolognia JL, Pawelek JM. Biology of hypopigmentation. J Am Acad Dermatol 1988;19:217-55.

Canizares O. Geographic dermatology: Mexico and Central America. Arch Dermatol 1960; 82: 870-93.

Carnevale A, Zavala C, Castillo VD, Maldonado RR, Tamayo L (1980) Analisis genetico de 127 families con vitiligo. Rev Invest Clin 32:37–41.

Casp CB. She JX. McCormack WT. Genes of the LMP/TAP cluster are associated with the human autoimmune disease vitiligo. Genes Immun 2003; 4: 492-9.

Cho S, Kang KC, Hahm JH. Characteristics of vitiligo in Korean children. Pediatr Dermatol 2000;17:189-93.

Das SK, Majumder PP, Chakraborty R, Majumdar TK, Haldar B. Studies on vitiligo. I. Epidemiological profile in Calcutta, India. Genet Epidemiol. 1985; 2(1):71-8.

Dawber RP. Vitiligo in Mature onset diabetes mellitus. Br J Dermatol 1968;80:275-8.

Deng GY. Muir A. Maclaren NK. She JX. Association of LMP2 and LMP7 genes within the major histocompatibility complex with insulin-dependent diabetes mellitus: population and family studies. Am J Hum Gen 1995; 56: 528-34.

El Mofty AM. Vitiligo and psoralens. Pergamon Press: Oxford; 1968. p. 1147-95.

El-Hazmi MA, Al-Swailem A R, Warsy A S, Al-Swailem A M, Sulaimani R, Al-Meshari A A. Consanguinity among the Saudi Arabian population. J Med Genet. 1995 August; 32(8): 623–6.

Engel L. What are those white patches in my patient's skin? Dermatol Nurs 2001;13:292-7.

Fain PR, Gowan K. LaBerge GS. Alkhateeb A. Stetler GL. Talbert J. Bennett DC. Spritz RA. A genome-wide screen for generalized vitiligo: confirmation of AIS1 on chromosome 1p31 and evidence for additional susceptibility loci. Am J Hum Gen 2003; 72: 1560-4.

Finco OM, Cuccia M, Martinetti G, Ruberto G, Orecchia G, Rabbiosi G. Age of onset in vitiligo: relationship with HLA supratypes. Clin Genet 1991; 39: 48-54.

Fitzpatrick TB. Phototherapy of vitiligo, in sunlight and man. Normal and abnormal biologic response. *In* : Pathak MA, editor. University of Tokyo Press: Tokyo; 1974. p. 783-91.

Fornara I. Quoted by Robert P. Uber die vitiligo. Dermatologica 1941;4:241-319.

Gauthier Y, Cario-Andre M, Lepreux S, Pain C, Taieb A. Melanocyte detachment after skin friction in non lesional skin of patients with generalized vitiligo. Br J Dermatol 2003;148:95-101.

Goudie BM, Wilkieson C, Goudie RB. A family study of vitiligo patterns. Scott Med J 1983; 28: 338-42.

Goudie BM, Wilkieson C, Goudie RB. Skin maps in vitiligo. Scott Med J 1983;28:343-6.

Grunnet I, Howitz J, Reymann F, Schwartz M. Vitiligo and pernicious anemia. Arch Dermatol 1970;101:82-5.

Hafez M, Sharaf L, El-Nabi SMA. The genetics of vitiligo. Acta Derm Venereol. 1983;63:249–51.

Halder R, Taliaferro S. Vitiligo. In: Wolff K, Goldsmith L, Katz S, Gilchrest B, Paller A, Lefell D, eds. *Fitzpatrick's Dermatology in General Medicine*. Vol 1. 7th ed. New York, NY: McGraw-Hill; 2008:72.

Halder RM. Childhood Vitiligo. Clin Dermatol 1997;15:899-906.

Handa S, Dogra S. Epidemiology of childhood vitiligo: A study of 625 patients from North India. Pediatr Dermatol 2003;20:207-10.

Handa S, Kaur I. Vitiligo - Clinical findings in 1436 patients. J Dermatol Tokyo 1999; 26: 653-7.

Hann SK, Lee HJ. Segmental vitiligo, clinical findings in 208 patients. J Am Acad Dermatol 1996;35:671-4.

Hann SK, Lee HJ. Segmental vitiligo: clinical findings in 208 patients. J Am Acad Dermatol 1996;35: 671-4.

Hann S-K, Nordlund J (2000) Vitiligo: a comprehensive monograph on basic and clinical science. Blackwell Science, Oxford, United Kingdom.

Hann SK, Park YK, Chun WH. Clinical feature of vitiligo. Clin Dermatol 1997;15:891-7.

Howitz J, Brodthagen H, Schwartz M, Thomsen K. Prevalence of vitiligo: Epidemiological survey the Isle of Bornholm, Denmark. Arch Dermatol 1977; 113: 47-52.

Jaigirdar MQ, Alam SM, Maidul AZ. Clinical presentation of vitiligo. Mymensingh Med J 2002;11:79-81.

Jeninger CK. Childhood vitiligo. Br J Dermatol 1993;51:25-8.

Kar PK. Vitiligo: A study of 120 cases. Indian J Dermatol Venereol Leprol 2001;67:302-4.

Khoo OT. Vitiligo. A review and report of treatment of 60 cases in the general hospital, Singapore, from 1954 to 1958. Singapore Med J 1962;3:157-68.

Kim SM, Chung HS, Hann SK. The genetics of vitiligo in Korean patients. Int J Dermatol. 1997;37:908–10.

Koranne RK, Sachdeva KG. Vitiligo. Int J Dermatol 1988;27:676-81.

Koranne RV, Sehgal VN, Sachdeva KG. Clinical profile of vitiligo in North India. Indian J Dermatol Venereol Leprol 1986;52:81-2.

Kovacs SO. Vitiligo. J Am Acad Dermatol 1998;38:647-66.

Le Poole C, Boissy RE. Vitiligo. Semin Cutan Med Surg 1997;16:3-14.

Le Poole IC. Sarangarajan R. Zhao Y. Stennett LS. Brown TL. Sheth P. Miki T. Boissy RE. VIT1, a novel gene associated with vitiligo. Pigment Cell Res 2001; 14: 475-84.

Lerner AB. Vitiligo. J Invest Dermatol 1959;32:285-310.

Lerner MR, Fitzpatrick TB, Halder RM, Hawk JL. Discussion of a case of vitiligo. Photodermatol Photoimmunol Photomed 1999;15:41-4.

Levai M. A study of certain contributory factors in the development of vitiligo in South Indian patients. AMA Arch Derm 1958;78:364-71.

Majumder PP, Das SK, Li CC. A genetical model for vitiligo. Am J Hum Genet. 1988;43:119–25.

Majumder PP, Nordlund JJ, Nath SK. Pattern of familial aggregation of vitiligo. *Arch Dermatol* 1993; 129: 994-8.

Majumder PP. Genetics and prevalence of vitiligo vulgaris. In: Hann SK, Nordlund JJ, editors. Vitiligo. Oxford: Blackwell Science; 2000. p. 18–20.

Mason CP and Gawk Rodger DJ (2005) Vitiligo presentation in adults. Clin Exp Dermatol. 2005 Jul; 30(4):344-5.

Mehta NR, Shah KC, Theodore C, Vyas VP, Patel AB (1973) Epidemiological study of vitiligo in Surat area. Indian J Med Res 61:145–154.

Moscher DB, Fitzpatrick TB, Hori Y, Ortonne JP. Disorders of pigmentation. *In* : Fitzpatick TB, Isen AZ, Wolff K, Freedberg IM, Austen KF, editors. Dermatology in general medicine. New York: McGraw Hill; 1993. p. 903.

Mosher DB, Fitzpatrick TB, Ortanne JB. Disorders of pigmentation, hypomelanoses and hypermelanoses, In: Freedberg IM, Eisen AZ, Fitzpatrick TB, editors. Dermatology in general medicine. 5th ed. New York: McGraw-Hill; 1999. p. 936–45.

Mosher DM, Fitzpatrick TB, et al. Disorders of pigmentation. In: Fitzpatrick TB, Eisen AZ, Wolft K, et al, editors. Dermatology in general medicine. New York: McGraw Hill Company, 1987;810-21.

Nath SK, Kelly JA, Namjou B, Lam T, Bruner GR, Scofield RH, Aston CE, Harley JB (2001) Evidence for a susceptibility gene, *SLEV1,* on chromosome 17p13 in families with vitiligo-related systemic lupus erythematosus. Am J Hum Genet 69:1401–1406.

Nath SK, Majumder PP, Nordlund JJ. Genetic epidemiology of vitiligo: multilocus recessivity cross-validated. Am J Hum Genet. 1994;55:981–90.

Njoo MD, Westerhof W. Vitiligo: Pathogenesis and treatment. AmJ Clin Dermatol 2001;2:167–181.

Nordlund JJ, Lerner AB. Vitiligo-it is important. Arch Dermatol 1982;118:5-8.

Nordlund JJ, Majumder PP. Recent investigations in vitiligo vulgaris. Dermatol Clin. 1997;15:69–78.

Ongenae K, Van Geel N, Naeyaert JM (2003) Evidence for an autoimmune pathogenesis of vitiligo. Pigment Cell Res 16:90–100

Onunu AN, Kubeyinje EP. Vitiligo in the Nigerian African: a study of 351 patients in Benin City, Nigeria. Int J Dermatol. 2003 Oct; 42(10):800-2.

Pajvani U, Ahmad N, Wiley A, Levy RM, Kundu R, Mancini AJ, Chamlin S, Wagner A, Paller AS. The relationship between family medical history and childhood vitiligo. J Am Acad Dermatol. 2006 Aug; 55(2):238-44.

Panja G. Leukoderma. Indian J Vener Dis 1947;13:56-63.

Perrot H. Vitiligo, Thyreopallisis et autominunization. Lyon. Med 1973;30:325-31.

Poojary SA. Vitiligo and associated autoimmune disorders: A retrospective hospital-based study in Mumbai, India. Allergol Immunopathol (madr) 2011 Apr 5. [Epub ahead of print].

Prahalad S. Kingsbury DJ. Griffin TA. Cooper BL. Glass DN. Maksymowych WP. Colbert RA. Polymorphism in the MHC- encoded LMP7 gene: association with JRA without functional significance for immunoproteasome assembly J Rheumatol 2001; 28: 2320-5.

Punshi SK, Thakre RD. Skin survey. Maharashtra Med J 1969;16: 535-6.

Ramaiah A, Mojamdar MV, Amarnath VM. Vitiligo in the SSK community of Bangalore. Indian JDermatol Veneroel Lepr 1988; 54: 251-4.

Rezaei N, Gavalas NG, Weetman AP et al. (2007) Autoimmunity as an aetiological factor in vitiligo. J Eur Acad Dermatol Venereol 21:865–76.

Ruiz-Maldonado R, Tamayo Sanchez L, Velazquez E. Epidemiology of skin diseases in 10,000 patients of pediatric age. Bol Med Hosp Infant Max 1977;34:137-61.

Sarin RC, Kumar AS. A clinical study of vitiligo. Indian J Dermatol Venereol Lepr 1977;83:190-194.

Sehgal VN. A clinical evaluation of 202 cases of Vitiligo. Cutis 1974;14:439-45.

Shah H, Mehta A, Astik B. Clinical and sociodemographic study of vitiligo. Indian J Dermatol Venereol Leprol 2008;74:701.

Shajil EM, Agrawal D, Vagadia K, Marfatia YS, Begum R. Vitiligo: Clinical profiles in Vadodara, Gujarat. Indian J Dermatol 2006;51:100-4.

Shwartz RA, Janniger CK. Vitiligo. Cutis 1997;60:239-44.

Singh M, Singh G, Kanwar AJ, Belhaj MS. Clinical pattern of vitiligo in Libya Int J Dermatol. 1985;24:233–5.

Spritz RA (2007). The genetics of generalized vitiligo and associated autoimmune diseases. Pigment Cell Res 20:271–8

Spritz RA (2008) The genetics of generalized vitiligo. Curr Dir Autoimmun 10:244–57.

Spritz RA, Gowan K, Bennett DC, Fain PR (2004) Novel vitiligo susceptibility loci on chromosomes 7 (*AIS2*) and 8 (*AIS3*), confirmation of *SLEV1* on chromosome 17, andtheir roles in an autoimmune diathesis. Am J Hum Genet 74:188–191.

Srivastava G. Vitiligo- Introduction Asian Clinic. Dermatol 1994;1:1-5.

Sun X, Xu A, Wei X, Ouyang J, Lu L, Chen M, Zhang D. Genetic epidemiology of vitiligo: a study of 815 probands and their families from south China. Int J Dermatol. 2006 Oct;45(10):1176–81.

Tawade YV, Parakh AP, Bharatia PR, Gokhale BB, Ran. Vitiligo : a study of 998 cases attending KEM Hospital in Pune. Indian J Dermatol Venereol Leprol 1997;63:95-8.

Tursen U. Kaya TI. Erdal ME. Derici E. Gunduz O. Ikizoglu G. Association between catechol-Omethyltransferase polymorphism and vitiligo. Arch Dermatol Res 2002; 294: 143-6.

Westerhof W, Bolhaar B, Menke HE, et al. Resultaten van een enquete onder vitiligo patienten. *Ned Tjdschr Dermatol Venereol* 1996;6:100–105.

Westerhof W. Vitiligo-a window in the darkness. Dermatology 1995;190:181-2.

Wittke-Thompson JK, Ambrose N, Yairi E et al. (2007) Genetic studies of stuttering in a founder population. J Fluency Disord 32:33–50

Wright AF, Carothers AD, Pirastu M (1999) Population choice in mapping genes for complex diseases. Nat Genet 23:397–404

Xu YY, Ye DQ, Tong ZC, Hao JH, Jin J, Shen SF, Li CR, Zhang XJ (2002) An epidemiological survey for four skin diseases in Anhui [In Chinese]. Chin J Dermatol 35:406–407.

Zaima H, Koga M. Clinical course of 44 cases of localized type vitiligo. J Dermatol 2002;29:15-9.

Zamani M, Spaepen M, Sghar SS, Huang C, Westerhof W, Nieuweboer-Krobotova L, Cassiman JJ. Linkage and association of HLA class II genes with vitiligo in a Dutch population. Br J Dermatol 2001; 145: 90-4.

Zeglaoui F, Souissi A, Ben Ayed A, Fazaa B, Kamoun MR. Epidemiological and clinical profile of vitiligo in Tunisia: retrospective study of 503 cases. Tunis Med. Dec; 85(12):1016-9.

Zhang XJ. Clinical profiles of vitiligo in China: an analysis of 3742 patients. Clin Exp Dermatol. 2005;30:327–31.

Zhang Z, Xu SX, Zhang FY, Yin XY, Yang S, Xiao FL, et al. The analysis of genetics and associated autoimmune diseases in Chinese vitiligo patients. Arch Dermatol Res. 2008 Oct 7.

2

The Pathogenesis of Vitiligo

Marlene Dytoc and Neel Malhotra
University of Alberta
Canada

1. Introduction

The question, "What causes vitiligo?" remains ambiguous. The lay population generally accepts that it is the concept of the "autoimmune destruction of pigment-producing cells called melanocytes" - however, this assertion has not been fully substantiated. The exact pathogenesis is unknown, but research shows that it is complex, involving the interplay of multiple factors, many of which are not elucidated. In the last century, much research has been dedicated to vitiligo and several overarching theories of its pathogenesis have emerged.

In addition to genetics, the Neural Theory was first proposed by Lerner *et al* in the 1950s (Lerner, 1959), and since then, the Autoimmune Theory, Reactive Oxygen Species Model and the Melanocytorrhagy Hypothesis have been developed.

2. The role of genetics in the pathogenesis of vitiligo

Numerous studies have investigated the effect genetics engender on the onset and development of vitiligo. It is important to recognize the patterns of vitiligo and its physical distribution, as the genetic basis for each type of distribution can differ. *Trichrome vitiligo* refers to lesions that appear white, light brown, and dark brown concurrently, with each color representing a stage of disease progression. *Inflammatory vitiligo* lesions present with pruritus and have elevated, erythematous margins. Distribution of the disease follows two basic patterns: *focal vitiligo* involves one or several macules at a single site, whereas *generalized vitiligo* (GV) involves a widespread and largely symmetrical distribution of macules. When GV becomes extensive, or coalesces to which point the vast majority of the body is involved and very few pigmented areas remain, it is deemed *vitiligo universalis*. Both focal and generalized types are considered *non-segmental vitiligo*, whereas *segmental vitiligo* refers to disease that occurs and remains stable in one unilateral region, but at the same time can be associated with lesions elsewhere (Wolff & Johnson, 2009).

2.1 Family-based studies and patterns of vitiligo inheritance

Studies demonstrate that a family history for vitiligo exists in 6.25-38% of patients (Njoo *et al.*, 2001); however, the exact mode of inheritance remains unclear (Njoo *et al.*, 2001). A study by Majumder *et al* (1988) suggested that recessive alleles at multiple unlinked loci interact epistatically to cause the vitiligo phenotype. They employed their own Multiple Recessive Homozygosis Model (Li, 1987) with a data set of 274 families that had one affected individual to develop this hypothesis (Majumder *et al*, 1988). The model assumes that vitiligo is a recessive trait, involving multiple, autosomal, and unlinked loci. After applying their population data to this model, they found no significant differences between the observed segregation probabilities and those calculated using the Multiple Recessive Homozygosis Model (1987). These results demonstrate that recessive alleles at multiple unlinked loci could be involved in the genetic pathogenesis of vitiligo.

Years later, researchers tested this hypothesis with another family-based study, gathering data on 194 affected families from the United States (Nath *et al.*, 1994). This study showed that approximately 20% of affected individuals, or "probands", had at least one first-degree relative also with vitiligo. After completing segregation analysis of their data, the researchers concluded that three epistatically interacting autosomal diallelic loci are involved, and individuals who maintain recessive homozygosity at these loci are affected by vitiligo (Nath *et al*, 1994).

A study examining 1,030 Korean vitiligo patients also demonstrated a clear pattern of familial aggregation. Of these patients, 120 had a family history of vitiligo and data from these patients was collected. They found clear father-to-son transmission in some families, effectively ruling out X-linked inheritance as a possible genetic etiology. If a threshold trait, in this case vitiligo, has a multifactorial mode of inheritance, its frequency in relatives of affected individuals approaches the square root of the trait's frequency in the general population. Using their data, they calculated that the threshold trait in first-degree relatives of vitiligo patients was similar to the square root of the trait's frequency in the general population. Thus, their findings suggest that the inheritance of vitiligo is polygenic (Kim *et al*, 1999).

2.2 Molecular genetics-based studies

Another group studied 102 families with more than one vitiligo-affected offspring (termed "multiplex" families) (Spritz *et al.*, 2004). Peripheral blood was collected, and genotyping was done on 660 people, and 300 were found to be affected with vitiligo. Following genome-wide linkage analysis of these individuals, and heterogeneity testing between families with autoimmune disorders and families with no history of autoimmune disorders, they concluded that, for generalized vitiligo, there are two phenotypic subcategories that involve different loci or alleles. For patients with vitiligo and other concomitant autoimmune diseases, associated loci include the auto-immune susceptibility (AIS)-1, AIS2 (on chromosome 7), and the systemic lupus erythematosus vitiligo-related gene (SLEV1, a locus on chromosome 17 that is detected in multiplex families with systemic lupus erythematosus). The other phenotypic category, involving patients with generalized vitiligo alone, is linked with the AIS3 locus (on chromosome 8) (Spritz *et al*, 2004).

In a study of 26 vitiligo patients from Jordan, researchers investigated NALP1 as a candidate gene for the pathogenesis of vitiligo (Alkhateeb *et al.*, 2010). NALP1 acts as a primary regulator of the innate immune system, primarily existing in Langerhans cells and T cells (Kummer 2007). Eight variants within the NALP1 genomic and promoter regions were genotyped and analyzed, of which two variants in the NALP1 promoter region (rs2670660 and rs1008588) were determined to have significant association with vitiligo and Caucasian patients. These results confirm findings by Jin *et al* in 2007 demonstrating the association between the single nucleotide polymorphism (SNP) rs2670660 and vitiligo in a Romanian population.

Another means of investigating the genetic basis of vitiligo predisposition is to carry out a genome-wide association study. Birlea *et al* (2011) used genotype data from 1,392 unrelated non-Hispanic white vitiligo patients and compared these to 2,629 non-Hispanic white controls to determine genetic associations with GV. Of the thirty-three candidate loci tested, only three (FOXP3, TSLP, and XBP1) had a primary association with GV. Whereas the exact function of genes TSLP and XBP1 are unknown, FOXP3 is known to be erroneous in the X-linked recessive multiple autoimmune disease syndrome. Further meta-analysis suggested XBP1 is the most significant GV susceptibility locus. Lastly, they determined that the locus CTLA4 maintains a secondary association with GV, having its primary association with the autoimmune diseases epidemiologically related to vitiligo (Birlea *et al*, 2011).

Other studies have gone beyond identifying what genes are involved, to the mechanisms behind how the expression of those genes may be modified in order to create the vitiligo phenotype. Deoxyribunucleic acid (DNA) methylation is an epigenetic process that plays a role in gene transcription and genomic imprinting, among other mechanisms (Li 2002 and Reik *et al.*, 2001). The methylation itself is carried out by enzymes called DNA methyltransferases (DNMT1, -3a, -3b). Zhao *et al* (2010) examined peripheral blood mononuclear cells (PBMCs) from vitiligo patients and controls, and measured messenger ribonucleic acid (mRNA) levels of DNMTs, methyl-DNA binding domain proteins (MBDs) and interleukin-10 (IL-10). Since IL-10 has been associated with autoimmune reactivity, and demonstrated to be sensitive to alterations in methylation status, its levels were also examined (Balasa *et al.*, 1998, Dong *et al.*, 2007, Szalmas *et al.*, 2008). In vitiligo PBMCs, it was found that methylation was increased in comparison with controls, and, notably, the methylation-sensitive region in IL-10 was hypermethylated. At the same time, IL-10 expression was significantly reduced in the vitiligo PBMCs. These results suggest that in vitiligo, changes in DNA methylation activity can alter the expression of genes involved in autoimmunity, thereby providing a potential means for creating the vitiligo phenotype.

In a similar way, Yun *et al* (2010) assessed genetic interactions by looking into the transforming growth factor beta-receptor II (TGFBR2). This receptor has immunologic signaling that may cause autoimmune disease through a variety of mechanisms including inhibition of inflammatory pathways and lymphocyte activation (Basak *et al*, 2009). This was performed on a Korean sample that consisted of 415 controls and 233 non-segmental vitiligo (NSV) patients that were genotyped. Following age and gender adjustments and data analysis, three SNPs for the receptor gene were found to be significantly associated with the NSV group, suggesting a possible role for TGFBR2 signaling in the pathogenesis of vitiligo.

The destruction of melanocytes results in the depigmentation observed in vitiligo. The ultraviolet radiation resistance-associated gene, or UVRAG, not only confers UV-damage resistance, but has also been demonstrated to play a role in autophagy – the process of cellular self-destruction that is potentially tied to autoimmune pathologies (Liang *et al.*, 2006). For these reasons, Jeong *et al* conducted a study to investigate a potential UVRAG association with NSV, or GV, in a Korean population. With 225 NSV patients and 439 controls, the researchers identified two SNPs of UVRAG that showed a significant genotype difference between the two groups, thereby suggesting a potential association between UVRAG and NSV (Jeong *et al.*, 2010).

Birlea *et al* (2010) did a genome-wide association study and located notable SNPs at 6q27. These SNPs were located near the insulin-dependent diabetes mellitus 8 locus (IDDM8), which is an association signal for type 1 diabetes and rheumatoid arthritis. In this study, 32 distantly related vitiligo patients from a Romanian founder population and 50 healthy controls from villages in its vicinity were genotyped. The region on 6q27 where the SNPs (specifically rs13208776) are located contains a single gene – SMOC2. This gene encodes a protein whose exact function is unknown, but it is postulated to be involved in growth and development (Liu *et al.*, 2009) and cell matrix interactions (Maier *et al.*, 2008).

Kingo *et al* (2006) have demonstrated that messenger ribonucleic acid (mRNA) expression of melanocyte proliferating gene 1, or MYG1 (a gene involved in early developmental processes), is elevated in lesional skin of vitiligo patients. Nine SNPs are found within the MYG1 locus for susceptibility to vitiligo (Philips *et al.*, 2010). The MYG1 gene consists of seven exons, culminating as 7.5 kilo-base pair (kb) of DNA on chromosome 12. In total, 10 SNPs are apparent within the gene. The study examined 124 unrelated Caucasian vitiligo patients in Estonia. The -119 promoter SNP demonstrated an association with vitiligo. Two alleles exist at this SNP, a more common -119C allele and a minor -119G allele. They found a higher frequency of the -119G allele in vitiligo patients compared to controls and that this increase was most prevalent in patients with active vitiligo. The Kingo *et al* (2006) study found that MYG1 expression was the same in non-lesional skin of non-active vitiligo patients and in control skin. In active vitiligo patients, MYG1 expression was increased in both lesional and non-lesional skin, and within the lesional skin of non-active vitiligo patients. These results taken together thus suggests that the -119G allele of the MYG1 promoter sequence is a potential risk-allele for developing vitiligo and for the active state of the disease (Philips *et al.*, 2010).

2.3 Studies involving the human leukocyte antigen

A Chinese study genotyped 1,178 vitiligo patients and 1,743 controls for any association HLA-DRB1*07 had with vitiligo, and found that the HLA-DRB1*07 positive group showed a significantly higher frequency of early age of onset, positive family history, and vitiligo-associated autoimmune diseases than that of the negative group (Hu *et al*, 2010). Another study examined the influence of HLA susceptibility on familial versus non-familial vitiligo. One hundred and fourteen patients were studied, of which 84 had a family history and 30 did not. Familial or not, the vitiligo patients demonstrated no significant difference in the type, stability, and severity of the disease. Both groups showed an increase in HLA alleles A2, A11, A31, A33, B17, B35, B40 and B44. Familial vitiligo was specifically associated with increased HLA A2, A28, A31 and B44. The study also demonstrated that vitiligo with onset at younger than 20 years old was correlated with increased numbers of HLA A2, A11, B17, B35 and B44 (Misri *et al*, 2009). The latter study suggests that the genetic pathogenesis of familial versus non-familial vitiligo is different, albeit possibly overlapping.

Ying *et al* (2010) conducted a study genotyping 579,146 SNPs in 1,514 GV patients and compared the results with control genotypes. Significant associations included SNPs of genes encoding MHC class I (between HLA-A and HCG9) and class II (between HLA-DRB1 and HLA-DQA1) proteins. SNPs of significance were found in genes related to other autoimmune diseases (PTPN22, LPP, IL2RA, UBASH3A, C1QTNF6). The SNPs of genes RERE and GZMB (both involved in immunity in general) (Ying *et al.*, 2010), and the TYR locus (which encodes tyrosinase, an enzyme required for melanogenesis) (Spritz *et al.*, 2003) were also important. Overall, these candidate associations with NSV support the assertion that NSV susceptibility loci are shared with loci associated with other autoimmune diseases (Ying *et al.*, 2010).

In another genome-wide association study, susceptibility loci were found on chromosome 6 and in the MHC (Quan *et al*, 2010). Genotyping of 6,623 vitiligo patients and 10,740 controls was carried out, and analyzed for 34 SNPs which deemed promising from a previous study. In the MHC region, two independent association signals were found (rs11966200 and rs9468925), the latter of which is potentially a novel HLA susceptibility allele. On chromosome 6, two significant SNPS were found at 6q27 in a block containing three separate genes. One of these genes, RNASET2, encodes a ribonuclease (RNAse). When this gene is overexpressed, it makes cells more vulnerable to oxidative stress (Thompson *et al.*, 2009), an important mechanism for melanocyte destruction. The two genes are FGFR10P, which encodes a fibroblast growth factor receptor and can play a role in cell cycle progression in some disorders (Acquaviva *et al.*, 2009), and the chemokine receptor 6 gene (CCR6) (Quan *et al*, 2010).

Another HLA-oriented study by de Castro *et al* (2010) examined the gene encoding the discoidin domain receptor 1 (DDR1). This gene encodes a tyrosine kinase receptor that affects cell differentiation, adhesion, and cytokine production (Yoshimura *et al.*, 2005). One of the three SNPs of DDR1 (rs2267641) was found to be significantly associated with vitiligo. No association with autoimmune disorders was observed in this study, which suggests that vitiligo susceptibility may or may not be aligned with autoimmune disease (de Castro *et al.*, 2010).

Thus, the genetics behind the pathogenesis of vitiligo appear multifactorial and causal associations are yet to be established.

3. The neural theory

3.1 Early development and important principles

Lerner's "Neural Theory" (1959) asserted that depigmentation in vitiligo results from increased discharge of a specific substance (*e.g.*, melatonin) at peripheral nerve endings in the skin; one that lightens pigment and discourages formation of new melanin. Lerner went on to report that many cases of segmental vitiligo followed a clear dermatomal pattern, and that vitiliginous lesions were found to exhibit hyperhidrosis at rest. His study of one hundred and twenty-eight vitiligo patients also found that 30% of patients reported significant emotional upset preceding onset of disease, and an additional 39% associated their onset with nervousness, accidents, illnesses, operations, or parturition. Overall, 69% patients associated vitiligo onset with stress (Lerner 1959).

To establish the role of stress and the onset of vitiligo, Manolache & Benea (2007) did a case control study with thirty-two vitiligo patients, forty-five alopecia areata patients, and controls suffering from skin disease clearly unrelated to stress (*e.g.*, infection). Data from vitiligo and alopecia areata patients were analyzed separately. Sixty-five percent of vitiligo patients noted stressful events at disease onset or exacerbation, compared to twenty-one percent of age and gender-matched controls. An odds ratio was calculated as 6.81 with a 95% confidence interval of 2.24-20.71. The majority of vitiligo patients reported their stressors were primarily associated with personal and financial issues. Overall, the study lends support to the notion that a stressful life event may contribute to the onset or exacerbation of vitiligo.

Koga & Tango (1988) described the clinical picture of vitiligo in 480 patients, and from their data they formulated a set of categories to better define the disease. *Type A vitiligo* is associated with autoimmune disease, halo-nevi, and the Koebner phenomenon. It can occur at any age, and it progresses continuously with periods of remission and exacerbation. On the other hand, *Type B vitiligo* has an early age of onset, and spreads rapidly for a short time and then ceases. More relevant to the neural hypothesis is *Type B vitiligo*, which spreads over an affected dermatomal area (Koga & Tango, 1988). An additional classification germane to the neural theory is segmental vitiligo, in which lesions occur in the distribution, or "segment" of one or more nerves, albeit not necessarily affecting the entire segmental region (Lerner 1959).

3.2 Histopathological, microscopic and ultrastructural studies

Al'Abadie *et al* (1995) used electron microscopy to examine nerve fibers in the superficial dermis from vitiligo and control patients. Biopsies were taken from marginal (*i.e.*, peripheral) and central areas of vitiligo lesions as well as non-lesional skin. Vitiligo patients consistently demonstrated significantly thicker Schwann cell basement membranes surrounding nerve fibers in both lesional and non-lesional vitiligo skin, compared to controls. Finally, nerve ultrastructure was not dependent on the location (marginal or central) of the vitiliginous lesion. These findings suggest that, although in vitiligo the ultrastructural changes of superficial nerves are subtle, there is neural involvement in the pathogenesis of vitiligo (Al'Abadie *et al.*, 1995).

Gokhale & Mehta (1983) further investigated the histopathology of skin from vitiligo patients. Their work examined the epidermis, dermal papillations, blood vessels, sweat glands, sweat ducts, hair follicles and sebaceous glands, dermal nerve and nerve endings, and the connective tissue of the dermis. Seventy-four patients were studied and researchers examined biopsies from depigmented areas and contralateral, pigmented areas from vitiligo patients and compared these with control biopsies from corresponding sites from unaffected individuals (Gokhale & Mehta, 1983). It was observed that more acute disease was associated with a high frequency of inflammatory changes and long-standing disease demonstrated significant degenerative changes in dermal nerves and sweat glands. The dermal nerves in 41% of patients were completely degenerated and 38% showed some degree of degeneration. Similar findings were present at the nerve endings. Gokhale & Mehta (1983) concluded that since melanocytes are of neural crest origin, the degeneration of dermal nerves and nerve endings could play a role in the development of vitiligo.

Another histological investigation searched for a relationship between vitiligo pathogenesis and Merkel cells, a type of neuroendocrine cell. These cells are localized to the epidermis and are more abundant in sun-exposed areas (Moll *et al.*, 1990, Lacour *et al.*, 1991). Moreover, these cells are continuous with nerve fibers. Bose investigated biopsies from five patients with stable vitiligo. Lesions and adjacent normal skin samples were compared to biopsies from unaffected control skin from normal subjects. All five patients had Type A vitiligo (*i.e.*, their lesions *did not* follow a strict dermatomal pattern). The monoclonal antibody TROMA 1 was used for indirect immunofluorescence study of the biopsies to detect the presence of Merkel cells. Bose (1994) found that in the adjacent normal skin biopsies of vitiligo patients, and in the normal skin biopsies of healthy controls, that TROMA 1 bound to an average of five Merkel cells on the basement membrane of hair follicles and skin. There was no binding of TROMA 1 to Merkel cells evident in lesional skin biopsies. Bose thereby observed the loss of Merkel cells in vitiliginous skin. Toxic metabolites resulting in melanocyte destruction could lead to the diminished number of Merkel cells, or an alternative mechanism may exist between melanocytes and Merkel cells that results in the loss of Merkel cells and eventually melanocyte loss.

3.3 The role of the sympathetic nervous system in depigmentation

The role of the sympathetic nervous system in tyrosinase activity and pigmentation was performed in an animal study. Laties and Lerner (1975) took twenty-eight brown-eyed, Dutch belted rabbits and resected the superior cervical ganglion on one side in 10, and interrupted the preganglionic nerve trunk in the remaining 18. Regardless of which sympathectomy procedure was used, the researchers considered signs of ptosis and miosis as indicators of successful surgical outcomes (*i.e.,* loss of sympathetic nervous system activity). They found that in all of the animals that survived longer than two months, the color of the eye ipsilateral to the surgery lightened compared to the other eye. The researchers also completed an assay for tyrosinase activity in the iris tissue and found that following both types of surgery, tyrosinase activity was diminished. This loss of enzyme activity could stop melanin production and result in depigmentation. This study suggests that there may be sympathetic nervous system dysfunction in vitiligo.

Wu *et* al (2000) sought to confirm whether the sympathetic nervous system was involved in the pathogenesis of vitiligo. They used laser Doppler flowmetry and iontophoresis to assess the level of microcirculation occurring in vitiligo lesions to in order to assess sympathetic nervous system activity. They examined ten patients with stable facial segmental-type vitiligo, and had two groups of controls. One control group contained ten stable non-segmental-type vitiligo patients, and the other control group had ten healthy, unaffected individuals. All patients were matched for age and gender, and "stable" was defined as no new lesions or changes in present lesions in at least 3 months. They found approximately three times the cutaneous blood flow on the lesional side compared to that of the contralateral normal skin in segmental vitiligo. No such differences were found in the non-segmental group, or the healthy controls. When the researchers administered sympathetic nervous system blockers (such as propranolol), the segmental type patients demonstrated a dramatic decrease in blood flow, whereas the other two groups did not. Notably, however, when the researchers measured baseline plasma levels of catecholamines (specifically adrenaline and noradrenaline), and adrenoceptor (alpha and beta) densities on blood cells, there were no significant differences across all three groups. Wu *et al.* contend that their results further support that the nervous system is indeed involved in the pathogenesis of vitiligo. In particular, they found that some level of sympathetic nerve dysfunction exists in segmental type vitiligo, and this possibly plays an important role in disease onset and progression.

3.4 Neuropeptide studies and neuronal marker investigations

Al'Abadie *et al* (1994) studied neuropeptides and neuronal markers in vitiligo patients. In 12 vitiligo patients and 7 unaffected control subjects, immunoreactivity for polyclonal general neuronal marker (PGP), calcitonin gene-related peptide (CGRP), vasoactive intestinal polypeptide (VIP), and neuropeptide Y (NPY) was tested. Compared to normal controls, nerve fibers reactive to NPY were increased in the marginal areas of lesions in half of the patients studied. In lesional biopsies, 25% of patients also showed increased reactivity for NPY compared to control subjects. Overall, there was locally increased NPY reactivity around blood vessels and in the dermis of lesions (predominantly in marginal biopsies). NPY is associated with noradrenaline in human dermal nerves and is known to potentially exert a local autonomic effect. Furthermore, it is also a potential modulator of the sympathetic response. These results suggest that changes in neuropeptide reactivity in vitiligo patients could be a factor in the onset or progression of the disease.

Lazarova *et al* (2000) carried out a similar study several years later. This study employed indirect immunofluorescence techniques to identify the immunoreactivity of nerve fiber endings in the skin to neuropeptides and found similar findingss as Al'Abadie *et al* reported in 1994. In affected skin samples, NPY was most intensely reactive; however, Lazarova *et al* found that CGRP was also increased, although not as significantly. Both studies suggest that neuropeptides play a role in vitiligo pathogenesis. Lazarova *et al* postulated that a precipitating factor, for example, stress, causes a significant secretion of neuropeptides like NPY, which subsequently set off other reactions that trigger the onset of vitiligo.

Furthermore, Yehuda *et al* (2005) examined the relationship between the neuronal marker NPY and stress in vitiligo. The trial included thirty-four male veterans, eleven of whom were not exposed to any military trauma, eleven exposed (to military trauma), veterans without post-traumatic stress disorder (PTSD), and twelve veterans who were exposed with PTSD. Plasma NPY levels were determined. Upon regression analysis of collected data, high NPY levels were associated with symptom recovery and effective coping with trauma or stress. This finding suggests that NPY may have a protective role in stress exposure.

Rateb *et al* (2004) studied the role of nerve growth factor (NGF), a neuropeptide hormone, in a cohort of 20 vitiligo patients and 10 non-vitiliginous control subjects. All but two vitiligo patients had widespread disease. NGF is an amino acid peptide hormone that is required for sympathetic nervous system function (Lewin *et al.*, 1996). Rateb *et al* (2004) measured NGF levels in the lesions and non-affected skin in vitiligo patients and in the skin of control subjects. They found significantly increased levels of NGF in the lesional skin of affected patients when compared to non-lesional and control skin. At the same time, NGF levels were still higher in the non-lesional skin of vitiligo patients when compared to control skin samples. Thus, NGF may play a neurochemical role in the pathogenesis of vitiligo, and its presence could be an important factor in the maintenance or destruction of melanocytes (David, 2001 as cited in Rateb *et al.*, 2004).

Peters *et al* (2004) investigated the role of NGF in stress-induced neurogenic inflammation using a mouse model in which mice were subjected to sonic stress and then examined for subsequent hair growth termination. Skin tissue NGF levels and NGF receptors TrkA and p75 neurotrophin receptor (p75NTR) were measured using fluorescence immunohistochemistry. They found that stress upregulates NGF expression in hair follicles. Stress also increased expression of the low affinity p75NTR NGF-receptor and decreased that of the high affinity TrkA receptor. Using retrograde tracing, the researchers also found that NGF injections, which mimic stress, increased the proportion of Substance P neurons in the dorsal root ganglia. Since Substance P is involved in neurogenic inflammation, their overall findings suggest that stress-induced NGF expression can set off neurogenic inflammation.

Another group of neuropeptides relevant to vitiligo includes catecholamines. Morrone *et al* (1992) measured catecholamine metabolite levels in the urine of vitiligo patients. The researchers argued that because many vitiligo patients associate their disease onset to a stressful event or injury, and that these situations often result in presynaptic release of catecholamines (namely dopamine, norepinephrine and epinephrine); therefore, catecholamines could play an important role in the pathogenesis of vitiligo. In particular, they measured the metabolites homovanillic acid (HVA), vanilmandelic acid (VMA), 3-methoxytyramine (MT), normetanephrine (NMN), metanephrine (MN), 3,4-dihydroxy mandelic acid (DOMAC), and 3,4-dihydroxy phenylacetic acid (DOPAC) in 24-hour urine samples. Their population included 150 patients and 50 healthy controls. Of the 150 patients, 15 had generalized vitiligo, 50 had segmental type, and 85 had acrofacial vitiligo. Three

groups were then created. Group 1 had 8 segmental and 18 acrofacial patients, all with early active phase (early onset) vitiligo or with disease progression (as indicated by number and size of lesions). The second group included patients who had no new lesions in the last 4-8 months (5 generalized, 10 segmental, and 19 acrofacial patients). The third and last group of patients had stable vitiligo lesions for 1-5 years. Twenty-four-hour urine collections from all groups showed that the first and second groups had HVA (a dopamine derivative) levels 4 to 10 times higher than controls, and VMA (an epinephrine and norepinephrine derivative) levels up to 3 times higher than controls. The long-term stable vitiligo patients showed no significant difference in any of the measured catecholamine metabolites when compared to controls. Overall, the results demonstrate that HVA and VMA urinary levels correspond to the onset and progressive active phases of vitiligo, regardless of the way the disease is distributed (segmental, generalized, or acrofacial). Morrone *et al* postulated from their results that the high urinary levels of HVA and VMA are markers of increased catecholamines in the circulation, and catecholamines are increased as a result of stress at the onset of disease. They also asserted that as patients grow accustomed to the lesions, their stress levels associated with the disease decreases, and consequently, so do levels of circulating catecholamines and urinary metabolites. This lends some support to the neural hypothesis, *i.e.*, that neurotransmitters may play a central role in the pathogenesis of vitiligo. They suggest that increased levels of catecholamines at autonomic nerve endings in the skin could be cytotoxic to melanocytes either directly or indirectly through their metabolites. Notable metabolites include melanotoxic phenols that can bind tyrosinase and interfere with melanogenesis. Morrone *et al* (1992) also suggested that stressful events could result in catecholamine discharge. These catecholamines could bind alpha-receptors in the skin and mucosa arterioles causing vasoconstriction, hypoxia, and overproduction of oxygen radicals that destroy melanocytes (Morrone *et al*, 1992).
The Neural Theory has been investigated internationally; however, substantial evidence supporting this has not yet been established. Mental stress can stimulate the secretion of catecholamines through stimulating the hypothalamic-pituitary-adrenal axis (Morrone *et al* 1992; Tolis & Stefanis, 1983; Stokes & Sikes, 1988). In addition, other neurogenic inflammatory mediators implicated in vitiligo pathogenesis, such as NPY (Ekblad *et al.*, 1984), NGF (Peters *et al.*, 2004), and NGF receptors (Tometten *et al.*, 2004) are also influenced by stress. These factors are postulated to result in melanocyte destruction via direct cytotoxic inflammatory or immune mechanisms. Therefore, pharmacologic agents and non-pharmacologic methods that alleviate mental stress and inhibit these neurogenic factors may be considered in the future as therapeutic targets for vitiligo.

4. The autoimmune hypothesis

As discussed previously, the neural hypothesis lends the most support for the pathogenesis of segmental-type vitiligo, whereas for non-segmental, or "generalized" vitiligo, the pathogenesis may be better explained by autoimmune mechanisms. One of the most apparent correlations between vitiligo and autoimmunity is the finding that patients with vitiligo often have autoimmune comorbidities. Another common finding in support of this hypothesis is that vitiligo often responds to immunosuppressive treatments (Lepe *et al.*, 2003). In this section, the pertinent research findings and arguments in support of the autoimmune theory of vitiligo pathogenesis will be discussed. The mechanisms of immunity are humoral (antibody-mediated), cell-mediated, or mediated by cytokines. Autoantibodies and their respective target cells are also relevant to the pathogenesis of vitiligo.

4.1 The role of autoantibodies, the humoral immune system and concomitant autoimmune disease

Kemp *et al* (2010) searched for autoantibodies against tyrosine hydroxylase (TH, an enzyme required for the production of catecholamine neurotransmitters) (Lewis *et al.*, 1993 as cited Kemp *et al.*, 2010). The researchers obtained sera from non-segmental vitiligo patients, 8 segmental patients, and 91 individuals with other autoimmune diseases (not including vitiligo), such as autoimmune thyroid disease, Addison's disease, and systemic lupus erythematosus (SLE). They also examined the sera of twenty-eight healthy controls with no history of autoimmune disease or vitiligo. Sera were tested for TH antibodies using a radioimmunoassay (RIA). They found that 23% of the patients with non-segmental vitiligo were positive for TH antibodies, whereas all control subjects and segmental-type patients were negative for TH antibodies. They also found a significant increase in TH positivity in patients with active disease over those with stable disease (defined here as no new or changing lesions in the previous 6 months). To confirm whether the TH antibodies were specific for TH, the researchers used absorption assays for several enzymes and found that the TH antibodies did not cross-react with phenylalanine hydroxylase (PAH) or tryptophan hydroxylase (TPH). Furthermore, in non-segmental patients, antibodies against MCHR1 (melanin-concentrating hormone receptor 1) and tyrosinase (Kemp *et al.*, 2010) were noted. These findings suggest autoimmunity plays a role in the development and activity level of non-segmental vitiligo.

Harning *et al* (1991) screened sera for antibodies against pigment cell-surface antigens and how their presence reflected vitiligo disease activity. Twenty-four vitiligo patients (10 with active and 14 with inactive disease), and nineteen healthy individuals who served as controls were included in this study. Active disease was defined as new or progressive disease within the 3 months prior to serum extraction. The researchers used a live-cell enzyme linked immunoabsorbant assay (ELISA) to detect relevant antibodies and their subtypes. They reported that the average level of pigment cell antibodies was notably greater in patients with active disease than in patients with inactive disease or in the controls, and there was no significant difference between inactive patients and controls. Results also indicated that immunoglobulin G (IgG)- and immunoglobulin M (IgM)-based pigment cell antibodies were found in 80% of active vitiligo patients. The control subjects and the inactive vitiligo patients demonstrated no IgG levels; however, 21% of inactive vitiligo patients and 16% of controls had notable levels of IgM. Immunoglobulin A (IgA) pigment cell antibodies were found in several individuals from the inactive and control groups - albeit in low levels (and the levels were not significantly different between these two groups). Harning *et al* demonstrate a relationship between pigment-cell antibody levels and vitiligo disease activity. This supports the idea that an autoimmune-mediated interaction with pigment cells exists in the pathogenesis of vitiligo.

As discussed earlier, vitiligo often occurs alongside other autoimmune disorders. Ingordo *et al* (2011) sought to decipher this relationship further by measuring circulating autoantibodies in a population of young southern Italian males. A total of 60 male vitiligo patients were included in the study. The average age was 19 years old, with an age range of 18-21. Circulating antibodies were found in 42.5% of these patients. Specifically, anti-thyroglobulin antibodies were detected in 27.5%, anti-thyroperoxidase in 22.5%, and anti-smooth muscle antibody in 17.3%. These antibodies are typically related to thyroid disease and other autoimmune diseases. They are of interest because vitiligo and thyroid disease are often associated with one another. In this study, only 5% of all patients presented with overt thyroid disease. Their results, when taken along with patient histories and analyzed using Fisher's exact test and T-testing, revealed that circulating autoantibodies, in particular anti-thyroid antibodies, were correlated only with recent onset of vitiligo. Their results showed that, in vitiligo patients, autoantibodies are often present without overt autoimmune disease, and that their presence, albeit related to onset, is unrelated to the course or extent of the vitiligo itself. Circulating autoantibodies thus may have an early role in the mechanisms ultimately leading to melanocyte destruction.

Similarly, Uncu *et al* (2011) examined the incidence of thyroid disorders in children with vitiligo using thyroid-specific tests. Fifty children with vitiligo (with an average age of 9.5 years, 26 males and 24 females) and fifty control children (25 males and 25 females, with an average age of 8.6 years and no history of autoimmune disorders) were examined for serum levels of free triiodothyronine, free thyroxine, (T3 and T4 respectively), TSH and antibodies to thyroperoxidase and thyroglobulin. All major subtypes of vitiligo were included in the patient population; however, generalized vitiligo was the most common. None of the subjects had overt thyroid disease; however 8% of the vitiligo group tested positive for autoimmune thyroiditis. No healthy controls were diagnosed with autoimmune thyroiditis. In addition, the researchers concluded that having concomitant autoimmune thyroiditis was more likely if the patient was female and if the duration of vitiligo was longer. This study further supports the association of vitiligo with autoimmune thyroid dysfunction, and that vitiligo may be caused by an autoimmune pathomechanism.

The humoral immune system likely plays roles in the autoimmune pathogenesis of vitiligo. The potential targets of these antibodies have been studied. A specific cell-surface target worthy of discussion is the melanin concentrating hormone receptor 1 (MCHR1). Using IgG from the sera of vitiligo patients and phage-display technology with a melanocyte complementary deoxyribonucleic acid (cDNA) phage-display library, Kemp *et al* (2002) first identified MCHR1 as a novel target for vitiligo autoantibodies in 2002. In total, 55 patients with vitiligo were enrolled, 41 with no autoimmune disorders, and 14 with one or more. Using radio-binding assays, immunoreactivity against MCHR1 was confirmed in sera from all of the patients. Antibodies to MCHR1 were found in 16.4% of the patients with vitiligo, whereas control sera exhibited no reactivity. Although this suggests that MCHR1 antibodies have a high disease-associated specificity for vitiligo, how they arise is unknown, and no obvious correlations between the presence of the antibodies and age of onset, gender, duration, subtype, or existence of concomitant autoimmune disease was determined. Normally, melanin concentrating hormone (MCH) binds MCHR1 (a G-protein-coupled receptor) to mobilize intracellular calcium (Chambers *et al.*, 1999) and acts as an antagonist of α-melanocyte-stimulating hormone (α-MSH). Studies by Hoogdijn *et al* (2001) suggest that MCH partially inhibits the induction of melanogenesis by α-MSH in human melanocytes (Hoogdijn *et al.*, as cited in Kemp *et al.*, 2002). Thus, signaling pathways involving MCHR1 could be involved in melanocyte regulation and melanin production (Kemp *et al.*, 2002).

Although MCHR1 was successfully identified as a target, how the antibodies interacted at this target was not elucidated. Gottumukkala *et al* (2006), sought to determine whether MCHR1 autoantibodies activate or block the MCHR1 response to MCH by studying nine vitiligo patients with MCHR-binding autoantibodies, nine vitiligo patients without these autoantibodies, ten patients with SLE (due to their tendency to exhibit notable autoantibody reactivity), and twenty healthy individuals ascontrols. IgG samples were taken from all participants, and fluorometry was used to detect intracellular calcium levels which would reflect MCHR1 activity. No control or SLE patient samples blocked MCHR1 receptor activity; however 56% of the IgG samples of vitiligo patients inhibited the function of MCHR1. No MCHR-activating autoantibodies were detected in any participant. The researchers found no correlation between the presence of MCHR-autoantibodies and vitiligo subtype, activity, age of onset, duration, or presence of concomitant autoimmune disease. This demonstrates that MCHR1-binding autoantibodies can block the function of MCHR1, and MCHR1 is a relevant B-cell auto-antigen in vitiligo (Gottumukkala *et al.*, 2006).

4.2 The role of cell-mediated immunity in vitiligo

Le Poole *et al* (1996) sought to elucidate what specific types of immune mechanisms were taking place in vitiligo. The perilesional skin of patients suffering from inflammatory vitiligo was evaluated. Inflammatory vitiligo is a relatively rare subtype of vitiligo in which perilesional skin is red, itchy, and irritated, and inflammation progresses outwards into unaffected skin. Consequently, the investigators hypothesized that the inflammatory process may play a role in the elimination of melanocytes. Thus, using antibodies, they examined the inflammatory infiltrates of the perilesional skin and determined their composition. Specifically, they used antibodies for melanocytes, T-cells (CD2, CD3, CD4, and CD8), Langerhans cells, and macrophages (CD36 and CD68). Each of these components was assessed immunohistologically by single and double immunostaining of the perilesional biopsies. Three inflammatory vitiligo patients were biopsied and results were compared to healthy control skin. The researchers found that melanocyte densities were 2.5 times greater in control skin than in the pigmented non-lesional skin of vitiligo patients. In perilesional skin, 66% of the patients demonstrated a marked decrease in melanocyte density when compared to non-lesional skin. CD3 staining of T cells was significantly greater in perilesional skin when compared to non-lesional or lesional skin. Also in perilesional skin, T cell infiltrates were substantially increased in the epidermal compartment and mostly concentrated to where melanocyte destruction occurs (at the epidermal basal layer). The epidermis-infiltrating T cells found in perilesional skin demonstrated an increased CD8:CD4 ratio, and increased interleukin-2 receptor (IL-2) expression. Interestingly, patients with generalized vitiligo have also been found to have an increased CD8:CD4 T cell ratio.

This finding suggests that the destruction of melanocytes could be cytotoxic CD8 T-cell mediated. All of the vitiligo patients also exhibited perilesional HLA-DR expression (MHC class II receptor), particularly along basal and suprabasal keratinocytes, which could be attributed to local T cell reactivity. Finally, Le Poole *et al* found that CD68+OKM5-type macrophages were more abundant in lesional and non-lesional skin when compared to controls, whereas the CD36 subset of macrophages were more abundant in control skin. From an autoimmune perspective, these results suggest that a melanocyte-specific immune reaction, most notably involving T cells, may play a role in the evolution of vitiligo.

4.3 The role of cytokines in vitligo

The immune system involves a complex interplay of many factors beyond lymphocytes and antibodies; this includes cytokines, which may also play a role in the development of vitiligo. Tacrolimus (FK-506 or Fujimycin) is an immunomodulatory drug thought to inhibit T cell activation and consequently diminish the production and secretion of pro-inflammatory cytokines (Schreiber & Crabtree, 1992 as cited in Grimes *et al.*, 2004). Grimes *et al.* (2004) performed a twenty-four week study that tested the effectiveness of 0.1%

tacrolimus ointment on nineteen patients with generalized vitiligo. The pre- and post-treatment cytokine expression in lesional and non-lesional skin compared to the expression in skin of normal controls was also assessed. A topical preparation of tacrolimus was applied twice daily for the 24-week study duration. Punch biopsies were performed at baseline from depigmented, non-sun-exposed lesional skin and adjacent non-lesional skin, and similar biopsies were taken from non-sun-exposed control skin. Following the 24-week treatment period, repeat biopsies were performed. A total of nineteen patients completed the study. Some level of repigmentation occurred in 89% of patients, most of which occurred in the face and neck regions. Overall, 68% of patients achieved between 76% and 100% repigmentation. In terms of cytokine expression, at baseline, both the involved and uninvolved skin of vitiligo patients demonstrated significantly increased expression of IL-10, IFN-γ, and TNF-α compared to expression in control skin. Post-treatment, the only significant difference was that expression of TNF-α was decreased compared to baseline in both lesional and non-lesional skin of the vitiligo patients.

These findings suggest that a cytokine imbalance is likely to be involved in the pathogenesis of vitiligo, and that the apparent suppression of TNF-α by tacrolimus may facilitate repigmentation. It is important to consider that repigmentation with tacrolimus was most notable in sun-exposed areas (*i.e.*, the face and neck). Therefore, it could be suggested that the suppression of cytokines, namely TNF-α, facilitates UV-stimulation of melanogenesis and ultimately, the repopulation of melanocytes in vitiliginous skin (Grimes *et al.*, 2003).

Considering that TNF- α and IFN- γ are both T helper cell-1 (Th1) cytokines, Taher *et al* (2006) suggest that vitiligo is mediated by the Th1 response. They also argue that tacrolimus could promote repigmentation by potentially suppressing the Th1 response via upregulating the immunosuppressive Th2 cytokine, IL-10 (Taher *et al.*, 2006). The researchers measured Th2-related cytokine IL-10 levels before and after treating twenty vitiligo patients with tacrolimus. Following three months of treatment, of the seventeen patients who completed the study, all experienced a significant decrease in lesion size, and all noted follicular repigmentation. On average, patients experienced a 41% decrease in the size of their lesions after the course of the treatment. In addition, IL-10 levels were significantly increased in lesional skin post-treatment, compared to normal control skin and lesional untreated skin. These results further supported tacrolimus as an effective vitiligo treatment. Bassiouny and Shaker (2011) further investigated the putative role of cytokines in vitiligo by studying interleukin 17 (IL-17). IL-17 is a cytokine that interacts with many cell types: keratinocytes, macrophages, and fibroblasts, amongst others. Furthermore, IL-17 works to activate the production of other cytokines, including IL-1 and IL-6, and can potentiate other local inflammatory mediators like TNF-α (Kolls & Linders, 2004, as cited in Bassiouny & Shaker, 2011). Using a similar ELISA technique as Harning *et al.*, the Bassiouny research team took a population of thirty patients with vitiligo and twenty healthy controls and examined their sera and tissue for the cytokine IL-17. They found increased levels of IL-17 in both the lesional skin and sera of the vitiligo patients, compared to that of the controls. In addition, they found a statistically significant positive correlation between disease duration and the level of IL-17 in both the sera and tissue samples. Although the exact function of IL-17 overexpression is unclear, this study affords further support for cytokine-involvement in the development of vitiligo (Bassiouny & Shaker, 2011).

The autoimmune hypothesis for vitiligo is has provided the basis for a vast number of experimental designs and studies. The immune system is complex, involving cell-mediated and humoral mechanisms - both of which appear to play roles in the manifestation of vitiligo. Identifying pathways involved in the immune reactions in vitiligo will help in understanding the cause of vitiligo and pave the way for developing specific immune targets to combat the disease.

5. The reactive oxygen species model

The theory that oxidative stress is a cause for vitiligo suggests that patients with vitiligo have an imbalanced redox (reduction-oxidation) state of the skin, resulting in the excess production of reactive oxygen species (ROS, *e.g.*, H_2O_2). These disturbances and ROS accumulation can have toxic effects on all components of the cell (*e.g.*, proteins, lipids), and could potentially result in the destruction of melanocytes creating the depigmented macules observed in vitiligo (Khan *et al.*, 2009).

5.1 Establishing the redox status of vitiligo patients

An early study relevant to this theory examined the anti-oxidant defense enzymes catalase (CAT), glutathione reductase (GR), and thioredoxin reductase (TR) in lesional and non-lesional skin using suction blisters from vitiligo patients (Schallreuter *et al.*, 1991). They found that TR levels were similar between patients and healthy controls; however, CAT levels were significantly decreased in both lesional and non-lesional skin of patients compared to healthy controls. Lastly, GR levels were also notably higher in patient skin compared to controls, with a significantly higher amount in the non-lesional, or pigmented skin of the patients compared to levels in the lesional skin. Since GR can facilitate some level of oxygen metabolism, the authors suggest that GR is upregulated as an attempt to compensate for the lack of catalase. Catalase is involved in oxygen metabolism, and these results suggest that catalase levels are decreased throughout the epidermis (spanning both affected and unaffected skin) in vitiligo patients. Thus, it is probable that oxygen metabolism is defective in vitiligo (Schallreuter *et al.*, 1991).

Ines *et al* (2006) examined the serum of thirty-six vitiligo patients (eighteen with stable and eighteen with active disease), and forty healthy controls for markers of redox status including malondialdehyde (MDA), selenium, vitamins E and A, and the erythrocyte activities of glutathione peroxidase (GPx), superoxide dismutase (SOD) and CAT. SOD scavenges superoxide radicals and reduces their toxicity (converts O_2^- to O_2 and H_2O_2) and catalase converts hydrogen peroxide (H_2O_2) to oxygen (O_2) and water (H_2O) (Ines *et al.*, 2006). MDA is a product of lipid peroxidation and is an indicator of oxidative stress (Latha & Babu, 2001, Yildirim *et al.*, 2004). Selenium is required for GPx activity and vitamins E and A are important in antioxidant activity. Ines *et al* found that SOD and MDA activity as well as serum selenium were increased in both stable and active disease, however, all were maximally increased in the active disease state. Erythrocyte CAT activity and serum vitamin A and E levels were not significantly different from controls. The researchers suggest that enhanced SOD activity results in the accumulation of H_2O_2. Furthermore, GPx is a downstream enzyme that detoxifies H_2O_2, and GPx levels were found to be decreased in vitiligo patients, which could compound H_2O_2 accumulation (Ines *et al.*, 2006).

Ines *et al* (2009) then sought to determine if disease activity was associated with oxidative stress at the tissue level. Tissue levels of MDA, CAT, SOD, and GPx from 10 stable and 10 active vitiligo patients were compared to levels found in twenty healthy volunteers. Overall, SOD, GPx, and MDA levels were all increased in both active and stable disease with consistently higher increases in the active group. Conversely, CAT activity was significantly decreased in both active and stable disease with a more notable decrease in the active group. This suggests that increased SOD activity in vitiligo patient tissue could be an adaptation to increased oxidative stress; however, the increased SOD ultimately results in H_2O_2 accumulation that can not be broken down by CAT because it is present in subnormal levels (Ines *et al.*, 2009).

Ines *et al* had some conflicting results between the 2006 and 2009 studies. The latter found decreased CAT levels and increased GPx levels in tissue, whereas previously, CAT was unchanged and GPx was decreased in patient serum. To substantiate the more recent Ines *et al* findings, Yildirim *et al* (2004) also found increased SOD, MDA, and GPx when examining the tissue of vitiligo patients. In addition, Khan *et al* (2009) found increased MDA, but significantly lower levels of SOD, GPx, and non-enzymatic antioxidant agents vitamins C and E in vitiligo patient serum. From these results, GPx is arguably increased in tissue, but its activity is decreased in the serum of vitiligo patients. The low SOD activity found by Khan *et al* is controversial, considering that the other studies discussed all found increased SOD activity. To reinforce this assertion, Sravani *et al* (2009) found statistically significant increases in SOD and CAT levels in both lesional and non-lesional skin of vitiligo patients compared to levels measured from skin from healthy controls. Furthermore, they found that CAT was decreased in both vitiligo skin typescompared to controls (Sravani *et al.*, 2009). Thus, the results from measuring similar markers vary somewhat from study to study. Khan *et al* suggested that these discrepancies could be due to differences between serum and tissue levels, duration, and activity of disease, as well as differences in laboratory techniques (Khan *et al.*, 2009). Nonetheless, when compared to controls, markers of oxidative stress in vitiligo patients are found at aberrant levels indicating that the balance between ROS and the anti-oxidant defense system is disrupted.

5.2 Characterizing the redox disruption in vitiligo

Dell'Anna *et al* (2001) suggested that the source of this disruption lies at the level of mitochondria. The research team retrieved and examined red blood cells (RBCs) and peripheral blood mononuclear cells (PBMCs) from forty non-segmental vitiligo patients and forty age- and sex-matched controls. They assessed the PBMCs for ROS generation using a 2′,7′-dichlorofluorescein diacetate (DCFH-DA) assay and flow cytometry analysis. They found significantly higher ROS generation in cells from active vitiligo subjects. Dell'Anna *et al* suggested that this ROS hyperproduction could be caused by opening of mitochondrial permeability transition pores (PTPs). They found that when they added a PTP inhibitor cyclosporin A, (CsA) to the cells, the DCFH-DA staining significantly decreased in the active vitiligo patients, reinforcing the notion that excess ROS production resulted from PTP opening at the level of mitochondria (Dell'Anna *et al.*, 2001).

To further characterize the redox imbalance in vitiligo and changes of mitochondria, blood samples were taken from fifty vitiligo patients (thirty-five with active and fifteen with stable vitiligo) and thirty healthy controls (Dell'Anna *et al.*, 2003). They measured the oxidative stress markers CAT, reduced glutathione (GSH), and SOD, and similar to previous research, found decreased CAT and GSH and increased SOD levels. Consequently, the SOD/CAT ratio was significantly higher in active disease and unchanged in stable and normal patients. ROS generation was significantly higher in active disease only. ROS levels correlated with the SOD/CAT ratio in controls and stable patients; however, the ratio was found to be inversely related to ROS activity in active patients. Thus, the researchers contend that excess

ROS production is an established phenomenon in vitiligo and when the disease is stable, this excess is balanced out by the body's cellular antioxidant system. Conversely, when the disease is active, and an oxidative stimulus is present, cells increase their ROS production and the redox balance is lost (Dell'Anna *et al.*, 2003).

In the same study, due to the function of mitochondria as the main intracellular source of ROS, mitochondrial function was also evaluated (Dell'Anna *et al.*, 2003). The researchers found a significant decrease in membrane potential across mitochondria in both active and stable vitiligo patients compared to controls. They also assessed the electron transport chain, or ETC, with a series of tests involving inhibitors of each complex. They found that PBMCs from vitiligo patients are susceptible to rotenone, an inhibitor of complex I. They also evaluated the Krebs cycle efficiency in mitochondria, and found the mitochondrial isoform of malate dehydrogenase activity was notably increased in vitiligo patients. These findings further support the assertion that mitochondrial dysfunction is involved in the pathogenesis of vitiligo (Dell'Anna *et al.*, 2003).

At the time, the cause of ETC impairment and mitochondrial dysfunction was yet to be elucidated. Thus, Dell'Anna *et al* investigated further using punch biopsies from five vitiligo patients and five healthy controls, and focused this study on characterizing lipid membranes. Confocal microscopy and fluorescence-activated cell sorting (FACS) revealed that epidermal primary vitiligo melanocytes had significant membrane peroxidation and that the pattern of fluorescence retrieved was specifically suggestive of the involvement of mitochondrial membranes (Dell'Anna *et al.*, 2007). To investigate the mitochondrial membrane changes more thoroughly, the content and transmembrane portion of cardiolipin, or CL was assessed. CL is a phospholipid that has four fatty acyl chains that is associated with mitochondria and with proteins that conduct oxidative phosphorylation (Haines & Dencher, 2002). There was a reduced percentage of CL and a modified distribution of CL in the melanocyte mitochondria of vitiligo patients, particularly in comparison with particulary in comparison with controls controls. Furthermore, to assess the ETC, they performed a semiquantitative analysis of complex 1 (CxI) activity and found CxI was decreased in melanocytes from vitiligo subjects when compared to the controls. These results provide a plausible mechanism for vitiligo pathogenesis in which there is a primitive defective arrangement of membrane lipids (namely altered CL distribution) that results in impaired ETC activity. Hyperproduction of ROS ensues, and the redox imbalance ultimately causes melanocytes destruction (Dell'Anna *et al.*, 2007).

5.3 The role of tetrahydrobiopterin recycling and other indicators of oxidative stress in vitiligo

The accumulation of hydrogen peroxide (H_2O_2) in the skin of vitiligo patients is an important finding, with many implications. One particular cellular pathway affected by H_2O_2 involves tetrahydrobiopterin. Tyrosinase is a hallmark enzyme in the synthesis of melanin (Prota, 1992). L-tyrosine is formed from L-phenylalanine by the enzyme phenylalanine hydroxylase (PAH). The essential cofactor for this process is 5,6,7,8-tetrahydrobiopterin or $6BH_4$. Defective recycling of $6BH_4$ yields excess levels of $7BH_4$, which is an inhibitor of PAH. This uncoupling of PAH and presence of $7BH_4$ was found in suction blister material from the skin of vitiligo patients (Schallreuter *et al.*, 1994, 1998). Kowlessur *et al* (1996) also found that $7BH_4$ production can lead to the formation of H_2O_2. To investigate this defective recycling of $6BH_4$ evident in vitiligo, Haase *et al* (2004) studied the enzyme dihydropteridine reductase, or DHPR, which is responsible for the final steps in normal $6BH_4$ recycling. They examined whole blood samples from twenty-seven untreated vitiligo patients and eight unaffected controls. The researchers also determined the effect of H_2O_2 concentration on DHPR activity. They found that concentrations of H_2O_2 greater than 30 μM decreased DHPR activity, whereas concentrations less than 30μM activated or increased DHPR activity. From this relationship it can be suggested that the accumulation of H_2O_2 through its concentration-dependent association with DHPR, results in defective $6BH_4$ recycling. They confirmed the concentration-dependent association between H_2O_2 and DHPR using Fourier transform-Raman spectroscopy. Interestingly, when patients were treated with topical pseudocatalase (low-dose narrow-band ultraviolet B-activated pseudocatalase PC-KUS – a treatment to remove epidermal H_2O_2), their whole blood DHPR activities normalized. This finding suggests that the removal of epidermal H_2O_2 affects systemic H_2O_2 balance. Overall, this illustrates the role ROS, namely H_2O_2, plays in the pathogenesis of vitiligo.

Schallreuter *et al* considered the effect of H_2O_2 on acetylcholinesterase (AchE). This enzyme was of interest because AchE levels were found to be lower in patients with vitiligo when compared with healthy controls, suggesting cholinergic involvement in the disease (Iyengar, 1989 as cited in Schallreuter *et al.*, 2004). Skin biopsies from sun-unexposed areas from four healthy controls and four vitiligo patients. Similar to the findings of Iyengar, Schallreuter *et al* found that depigmented vitiligo skin showed marked decreases in AchE levels compared to controls while repigmenting patients treated with PC-KUS demonstrated an increase in AchE throughout the epidermis. Untreated depigmented skin showed very little catalase activity, and PC-KUS-treated skin showed significantly higher catalase expression throughout the epidermis compared to controls. Thus, H_2O_2 levels were also found to have a concentration-dependent influence on AchE, *i.e.*, low H_2O_2 concentrations (approximately 10^{-6}M or mol/L) activate AchE whereas high concentrations (10^{-3}M or mol/L) deactivate AchE (Schallreuter *et al.*, 2004). Butyrylcholinesterase (BchE) is an enzyme that mediates the hydrolysis of acetylcholine. The hydrolysis reaction is one of the rate-limiting steps in cholinergic signal transduction (Rakonczay & Brimijoin, 1988 as cited in Schallreuter *et al.*, 2006). Using immunofluorescence, Schallreuter *et al* (2006) demonstrated that BchE is present in the keratinocytes and melanocytes of the human epidermis; however the BchE protein is much lower in skin from vitiligo patients. Upon removal of epidermal H_2O_2 using PC-KUS, vitiligo patient skin demonstrated a higher level of BchE expression than controls. When AchE and BchE activities were tested at the same time on the same samples, BchE activity levels were greater than the AchE levels. The overall decreased activities of BchE and AchE were apparent in both lesional and non-lesional skin of vitiligo patients demonstrating that the effects of H_2O_2 occur throughout the entire epidermal compartment.

Considering the previous research on H_2O_2 accumulation in vitiligo, Shalbaf *et al* (2008) investigated xanthine oxidase (XO) as a source of H_2O_2 because it produces H_2O_2 in its reaction pathway. XO is found in many tissues and catalyzes the oxidative hydroxylation of hypoxanthine to xanthine and then xanthine to uric acid, which is accompanied by H_2O_2 production (Mathews *et al.*, 2000 as cited in Shalbaf *et al.*, 2008). XO also oxidizes uric acid to allantoin, a substance that acts a marker of oxidative stress (Benzie *et al.*, 1999). Using skin biopsies from vitiligo patients, the presence of XO was confirmed in melanocytes and keratinocytes, and regulation of XO by H_2O_2 was also confirmed; high concentrations of H_2O_2 inhibit the activity of XO, whereas low concentrations activate it, making the relationship concentration-dependent. Epidermal cell extracts from suction blister tissue showed that allantoin was present in patients with acute vitiligo; however, it was entirely absent in healthy controls. Thus, XO may be a contributor of H_2O_2 ROS in vitiligo.

The vast majority of studies germane to the ROS model recruited patients with generalized vitiligo, and ROS-mediated damage may be applied to the pathogenesis of non-segmental, generalized vitiligo until further research is done in other types of vitiligo.

6. The melanocytorrhagy hypothesis

Compared to the other hypotheses discussed, the melanocytorrhagy hypothesis is a relatively new approach to explaining the pathogenesis of vitiligo. First proposed by Gauthier *et al* in 2003, this theory describes the pathogenesis of non-segmental vitiligo (NSV) as from the result of "melanocytorrhagy", or a chronic detachment and loss of melanocytes resulting from altered melanocytes responses to trauma and other stressors. The theory also attempts to tie together concepts from the theories previously discussed to create a single, integrated explanation of vitiligo pathogenesis, and suggests that stressors could include catecholamines, ROS, or autoimmune elements (Gauthier *et al.*, 2003).

Early studies by Le Poole *et al* demonstrated that melanocytes loss occurs in vitiligo lesions (Le Poole *et al.*, 1993). Gauthier *et al* countered that although melanocyte loss is well-established, direct demonstration of the physical destruction of melanocytes is not.

A study supporting the concept of melanocyte loss in vitiligo was done by Tobin *et al* in 2000. Twenty-seven patients with non-segmental vitiligo and ten healthy controls were enrolled. Seven patients received pseudocatalase treatment prior to the study, whereas twenty had received no previous treatment. The researchers acquired epidermal melanocytes and keratinocyte cultures from both lesional and non-lesional skin from vitiligo patients and normal controls. Light and transmission electron microscopy, as well as immunohistochemistry were used to evaluate the cultures for morphology. In the untreated vitiligo patient samples, they found vacuolation and degeneration of basal keratinocytes, melanocytes, and Langerhans cells. Also observed was an increased number of Langerhans cells in the basal layer of the epidermis near dysfunctional melanocytes, and dilated endoplasmic reticulum, intracellular granular debris, and fatty degeneration. Tobin *et al* attributed these changes to the oxidative stress caused by H_2O_2.

More importantly, there were signs suggesting melanocytes were never entirely absent. Evidence of rare clear cells in the epidermis of lesional skin from vitiligo patients with disease duration of up to twenty-five years was observed. These cells were small and amelanotic, although a portion of the clear cells did contain irregular melanosomes. These clear cells were deemed melanocytic as they contained tyrosinase (due to positive dopa reactivity). Although these cells were in significantly low numbers, these findings suggest that melanocytes are not entirely eliminated from vitiliginous skin and that they persist in some form, even in long-standing disease (Tobin *et al.*, 2000).

Gauthier *et al* (2003) also purports that defective cell adhesion plays a role in the pathogenesis of vitiligo as the production extracellular matrix components may be altered by keratinocytes. Basal membrane structure dysfunction is observed in vitiligo, in particular, the presence of focal gaps in the basement membrane and redundant production of basement membrane. These alterations could weaken the basal anchoring of melanocytes, making them vulnerable to detachment. Trauma could exacerbate this vulnerability, leading to the chronic melanocyte loss that has been described as melanocytorrhagy.

Le Poole *et al* argued that the protein tenascin may be involved in diminishing melanocyte adhesion in the pathogenesis of vitiligo. Skin biopsies of lesional and control skin were examined. In normal culture conditions, melanocytes most easily adhere to the extracellular matrix (ECM) protein fibronectin. There was an observed relationship between tenascin concentration and melanocyte adhesiveness to fibronectin: an abundance of tenascin inhibited melanocyte to fibronectin adhesion. In general, the vitiligo patients were found to express higher levels of tenascin compared to controls. Whether the increased tenascin expression is a cause or consequence of vitiligo is unclear; however, from these results it is arguable that modified cellular adhesion is evident in vitiligo and could contribute to its pathogenesis (Le Poole *et al.*, 1997).

A pivotal study regarding the melanocytorrhagy hypothesis investigated how trauma could elicit vitiligo lesions, a process also called the Koebner phenomenon. Light and reproducible friction for four minutes on the forearms of eighteen patients with extensive vitiligo and on five healthy controls was performed. Biopsies were retrieved from the test region from all sets of patients at 1, 4, 24, and 48 hours after the friction was imposed. Each biopsy was evaluated using standard light microscopy, transmission electron microscopy, histochemistry, and immunohistochemistry. Control skin showed no changes; however, at 4 and 24 hours post-friction in vitiliginous skin, some melanocytes were detached and apparent in suprabasal regions, *i.e.,* the stratum spinosum, granular layer, and the stratum corneum. The researchers thought that vitiligo arising from the Koebner phenomenon is likely caused by the "transepidermal migration" observed in their study. They also concluded that this mechanism of melanocyte loss could provide an explanation for the chronic melanocyte loss evident in vitiligo, but may be instigated by another stressor other than friction or trauma (Gauthier *et al.*, 2003).

The melanocytorrhagy hypothesis was tested by recreating the initiating events leading up to melanocytorrhagy (Cario-André *et al.*, 2007). Epidermis was reconstructed on dead de-epidermized dermis (DDD) using control cells and cells from non-lesional NSV patients to form "new" epidermis. Since the "new" epidermis was weakly attached to the DDD, it was assumed that physical friction would not be required to initiate melanocytorrhagy. The reconstructs were subject to a variety of stressors, for example, epinephrine, norepinephrine, and H_2O_2. Reconstructs made with non-lesional vitiligo melanocytes had fewer basal melanocytes when compared to reconstructs made with normal melanocytes, suggesting that non-lesional NSV skin is affected by the disease process.

The reconstructs from vitiligo patients and found that 65% of the sera samples tested were able to induce melanocyte detachment. Epinephrine was also found to cause melanocyte detachment of normal and non-lesional vitiligo melanocytes; however norepinephrine had no effect on detachment at any concentration. Furthermore, H2O2 caused normal melanocyte…" (add space between H2O2 and caused) detachment, with variable effects on non-lesional vitiligo melanocytes. An intrinsic melanocyte defect limits melanocyte adhesion in reconstructed epidermis, and transepidermal migration melanocytes can occur in response to certain stressors (Cario-André *et al.*, 2007). Although an early *in vitro* study, these results provide some support for the melanocytorrhagy model.

Gauthier *et al* also indirectly support this theory in their early research. Their findings show that chronic melanocyte loss and defective adhesion could be the result of the dendritic function of melanocytes. Melanocyte dendrites are thought to be required for melanosome transfer as these processes connect melanocytes to numerous keratinocytes. Dendrites may play a role in melanocyte adhesion and anchoring within the basal layer of the epidermis, and dendrite retraction is commonly understood as the first step before melanocyte detachment and death. Morphologically, established vitiligo melanocytes demonstrate large perikaryon and "stubby" dendrites (Jimbow *et al.*, 2000). Exposing cultures of vitiligo or control melanocytes to catecholamines could result in dendrite retraction and loss over a twenty-four hour period. Consequently, the research group concluded that oxyradicals or catecholamines could cause dendrite loss, thereby compounding the transepidermal melanocyte loss caused by an isomorphic or the Koebner phenomenon, resulting in the depigmented macules observed in vitiligo.

The melanocytorrhagy theory for the pathogenesis of vitiligo takes a new stance on how melanocyte loss occurs, and attempts to unify ideas from several pathogenesis theories to do so. Being a novel proposal, however, further research is needed to substantiate its postulations.

7. Conclusion

The pathogenesis of vitiligo has yet to be elucidated; however, years of research have provided us with a framework. A genetic predisposition to developing the disease is involved. The Neural Hypothesis suggests that the nervous system is involved, likely through the release of neurogenic factors in response to a stress event, and that these factors affect the survival of melanocytes. Cytotoxic and immune mechanisms are proposed to underlie the destruction of melanocytes through neuropeptides. The Autoimmune Theory argues that the loss of melanocytes observed in vitiligo is the result of an autoimmune reaction. The Reactive Oxygen Species Model suggests that faulty oxygen metabolism results in the excess production of reactive oxygen species, which causes melanocyte destruction. In addition, the Melanocytorrhagy Theory states that melanocyte loss occurs from defective cell adhesion coupled with friction or other types of stress. These mechanisms underlying vitiligo pathogenesis likely overlap and may vary depending on the type of vitiligo. Genetic factors likely precede neurogenic factors which, influenced by mental stress, may act via the aforementioned cytotoxic and immune mechanisms to cause destruction of melanocytes and resulting skin depigmentation. Future research would elucidate if these theories occur in a sequential fashion. Strategies targeting these pathways would potentially advance our therapeutic armament against vitiligo.

8. References

Acquaviva, C., Chevrier, V., Chauvin, JP *et al.* (2009). The centrosomal FOP protein is required for cell cycle progression and survival. *Cell Cycle*, Vol. 8, No. 8, (Apr 2009), pp.1217-27, 1551-4005

Al'Abadie, MSK., Senior, HJ., Bleehen, SS., *et al.* (1994). Neuropeptide and neuronal marker studies in vitiligo. *British Journal of Dermatology*, Vol. 131, No. 2, (Aug 1994), pp.160-165, 0007-0963

Alkhateeb, A., Qaraz, F. (2010). Genetic association of NALP1 with generalized vitiligo in Jordanian Arabs. *Archives of Dermatology Research*, Vol. 302, No. 8, (Oct 2010), pp. 631-634, 0340-3696

Basak, PY., Adiloglu, AK, Ceyhan, AM *et al.* (2009). The role of helper and regulatory T cells in the pathogenesis of vitiligo. *Journal of American Academy of Dermatology*, Vol. 60, No.2, (Feb 2009), pp.256-60, 0190-9622

Bassiouny, DA., & Shaker, O. (2011). Role of interleukin-17 in the pathogenesis of vitiligo. *Clinical and Experimental Dermatology*, Vol. 36, No. 3, (Apr 2011), pp.292-297, 1365-2230

Benzie, IFF., Chung, WY., Tomlinson, B. (1999). Simultaneous Measurement of Allantoin and Urate in Plasma: Analytical Evaluation and Potential Clincial Application in

Oxidant:Antioxidant Balance Studies. *Clinical Chemistry*, Vol. 35, No. 6, (Jun 1999), pp.901-4

Birlea, SA., Gowan, K., Fain, PR *et al.* (2010). Genome-Wide Association Study of Generalized Vitiligo in an Isolated European Founder Popoulation Identifies SMOC2, in Close Proximity to IDDM8. *Journal of Investigative Dermatology*, Vol. 130, No. 3 (Mar 2010), pp.798-803

Birlea, SA., Jin, Y., Bennett, DC *et al.* (2011). Comprehensive Association Analysis of Candidate Genes for Generalized Vitiligo Supports XBP1, FOXP3, and TSLP. *Journal of Investigative Dermatology*, Vol. 131, No. 2, (Feb 2011), pp.371-381, 1523-1747

Bose, SK. (1994). Probable mechanisms of loss of Merkel cells in completely depigmented skin of stable vitiligo. *The Journal of Dermatology*, Vol. 21, No. 10, (Oct 1994), pp.725-8, 0385-2407

Cario-Andre, M., Pain, C., Gauthier, Y., *et al.* (2007). The melanocytorrhagic hypothesis of vitiligo tested on pigmented, stressed, reconstructed epidermis. *Pigment Cell Research*, Vol. 20, No. 5, (Oct 2007), pp.385-393, 0893-5785

Chambers, J., Ames, RS., Bergsma, D., *et al.* (1999). Melanin-concentrating hormone is the cognate ligand for the orphan G-protein-coupled receptor SLC-1. *Nature*, Vol. 400, No. 6741, (Jul 1999), pp.261-265, 0028-0836

David, A. (2001). The neurosensory system controls keratinocyte release of growth and survival factor nerve growth factor. *Journal of Investigative Dermatology*, Vol. 117, No. 5, pp.1025

De Castro, CCS., do Nascimento, LM., Walker, G *et al.* (2010). Genetic Variants of the DDR1 Gene Are Associated with Vitiligo in Two Independent Brazilian Population Samples. *The Society for Investigative Dermatology*, Vol. 130, No. 7, (Jul 2010), pp.1813-18, 1523-1747

Dell'Anna, ML., Maresca,V., Briganti, S., *et al.* (2001). Mitochondrial Impairment in Peripheral Blood Mononuclear Cells During the Active Phase of Vitiligo. *Journal of Investigative Dermatology*, Vol. 117, No. 4, (Oct 2001), pp.908-913, 0022-202X

Dell'Anna, ML., Ottaviani, M., Albanesi, V., *et al.* (2007). Membrane Lipid Alterations as a Possible Basis for Melanocyte Degeneration in Vitiligo. *Journal of Investigative Dermatology*, Vol. 127, No. 5, (May 2007), pp.1226-1233, 0022-202X

Dell'Anna, ML., Urbanelli, S., Mastrofrancesco, A., *et al.* (2003). Alterations of Mitochondria in Peripheral Blood Mononuclear Cells of Vitiligo Patients. *Pigment Cell Research*, Vol. 16, No. 5, (Oct 2003), pp.553-559, 0893-5785

Ekblad, E., Edvinsson, L., Wahlestedt, C., *et al.* (1984). Neuropeptide Y co-exists and co-operates with noradrenaline in perivascular nerve fibers. *Regulatory Peptides*, Vol. 8, No. 3, (Apr 1984), pp.225-235, 0167-0115

Gauthier, Y., Cario-Andre, M., Lepreux, S., *et al.* (2003). Melanocyte detachment after skin friction in non-lesional skin of patients with generalized vitiligo. *British Journal of Dermatology*, Vol. 148, No. 1, (Jan 2003), pp.95-101, 0007-0963

Gauthier, Y., Cario-Andre, M., Taieb, A. (2003). A Critical Appraisal of Vitiligo Etiologic Theories. Is Melanocyte Loss a Melanocytorrhagy? *Pigment Cell Research*, Vol. 16, No. 4, (Aug 2003), pp.322-332, 0893-5785

Gokhale, BB., Mehta, LN. (1983). Histopathology of Vitiliginous Skin. *International Journal of Dermatology*, Vol. 22, No. 8 (Oct 1983), pp.477-80, 0011-9059

Gottumukkala, RSRK., Gavalas, NG., Akhtar, S., *et al.* (2006). Function-blocking autoantibodies to the melanin-concentrating hormone receptor in vitiligo patients. *Laboratory Investigation*, Vol. 86, No. 8, (Aug 2006), pp.781-789, 0023-6837

Grimes, PE., Morris, R., Avaniss-Aghajani, E., *et al.* (2004). Topical tacrolimus therapy for vitiligo: Therapeutic responses and skin messenger RNA expression of proinflammatory cytokines. *Journal of American Dermatology*, Vol. 51, No. 1, (Jul 2004), pp.52-61, 1097-6787

Haines, TH., & Dencher, NA. (2002). Cardiolipin: a proton trap for oxidative phosphorylation. *Federation of European Biochemical Sciences*, Vol. 528, No. 1-3, (Sept 2002), pp.35-39, 0014-5793

Harning, R., Cui, J., Bystryn, JC. (1991). Relation Between the Incidence and Level of Pigment Cell Antibodies and Disease Activity in Vitiligo. *The Society for Investigative Dermatology*, Vol. 97, No. 6, (Dec 1991), pp.1078-80, 0022-202X

Haase, S., Gibbons, NCJ., Rokos, H., *et al.* (2004). Perturbed 6-Tetrahydrobiopterin Recycling via Decreased Dihydropteridine Reductase in Vitiligo: More Evidence for H_2O_2 Stress. *Journal of Investigative Dermatology*, Vol. 122, No. 2, (Feb 2004), pp.307-313, 0022-202X

Hoogdijn, MJ., Ancans J., & Thody, AJ. (2001). Melanin-concentrating hormone may act as a paracrine inhibitor of melanogenesis. *British Journal of Dermatology*, Vol. 144, pp.651-677, ISSN

Hu, DY., Ren, YQ., Zhu, KJ *et al.* (2011). Comparisons of clinical features of HLA-DRB1*07 positive and negative vitiligo patients in Chinese Han population. *Journal of the European Academy of Dermatology and Venereology*, (Jan 2011)

Ines, D., Boudaya, S., Abdallah, FB., *et al.* (2009). Antioxidant enzymes and lipid peroxidation at the tissue level in patients with stable and active vitiligo. *International Journal of Dermatology*, Vol. 48, No. 5, (May 2009), pp.476-480, 1365-4632

Ines, D., Boudaya, S., Riadh, BM., *et al.* (2006). A comparative study of oxidant-antioxidant status in stable and active vitiligo patients. *Archives of Dermatological Research*, Vol. 298, No. 4, (Sept. 2006), pp.147-152, 0340-3696

Ingordo, V., Gentile, C., Iannazzone, SS., *et al.* (2010). Vitiligo and autoimmunity: an epidemiological study in a representative sample of young Italian males. *Journal of the European Academy of Dermatology and Venereology*, Vol. 25, No. 1, (Jan 2011), pp.105-109, 1648-3083

Iyengar, B. (1989). Modulation of melanocyte activity by acetylcholine. *Acta Anatomica*, Vol. 36, No. 32 (1989), pp.139-141

Jeong, TJ., Shin, MK., Uhm, YK *et al.* (2010). Association of UVRAG polymorphisms with susceptibility to non-segmental vitiligo in a Korean sample. *Experimental Dermatology*, Vol. 19, No. 8, (Aug 2010), pp.323-5, 1600-0625

Jimbow, K., Chen, H., Park, JS., *et al.* (2001). Increased sensitivity of melanocytes to oxidative stress and abnormal expression of tyrosinase-related protein in vitiligo. *British Journal of Dermatology*, Vol. 144, No. 1, (Jan 2001), pp.55-65, 0007-0963

Jin, Y., Birlea, SA., Fain, PR., *et al.* (2007). Genetic Variations in NALP1 are Associated with Generalized Vitiligo in a Romanian Population. *Journal of Investigative Dermatology*, Vol. 127, No. 11, (Nov 2007), pp.2558-2562, 1523-1747

Jin, Y., Birlea, SA., Fain, PR *et al.* (2010). Variant of TYR and Autoimmunity Susceptibility Loci in Generalized Vitiligo. *The new England Journal of Medicine*, Vol. 362, No. 18, (May 2010), pp.1686-97, 1533-4406

Kemp, HE., Emhemad, S., Akhtar, S., *et al.* (2010). Autoantibodies against tyrosine hydroxylase in patients with non-segmental (generalised) vitiligo. *Experimental Dermatology*, Vol. 20, No. 1, (Jan 2011), pp.35-40, 1600-0625

Kemp, HE., Waterman, EA, Hawes, BE., *et al.* (2002). The melanin-concentrating hormone receptor 1, a novel target of autoantibody responses in vitiligo. *The Journal of Clinical Investigation*, Vol. 109, No. 7, (Apr 2002), pp.923-930, 0021-9738

Khan, R., Satyam, A., Gupta, S., *et al.* (2009). Circulatory levels of antioxidants and lipid peroxidation in Indian patients with generalized and localized vitiligo. *Archives of Dermatological Research*, Vol. 301, No. 10 (Oct 2009), pp.731-737, 1432-069X

Kim, SM., Chung, HS., Hann, SK., (1999). The genetics of vitiligo in Korean patients. *International Journal of Dermatology*, Vol. 37, No. 12, (Dec 1998), pp.908-10, 0011-9059

Kingo, K., Philips, MA., Aunin, E *et al.* (2006). MYG1, novel melanocyte related gene, has elevated expression in vitiligo. *Journal of Dermatological Science*, Vol. 44, No. 2, (Nov 2006), pp.119-122, 0923-1811

Koga, M., & Tango, T. (1988). Clinical features and course of type A and type B vitiligo. *British Journal of Dermatology*, Vol. 118, No. 2, (Feb 1988), pp. 223-228, 0007-0963

Kolls, JK., & Linders, A. (2004). Interleukin-17 Family Members and Inflammation. *Immunity*, Vol. 21, No. 4, (Oct 2004), pp.467-476, 1074-7613

Kowlessur, D., Citron, BA., Kaufman, S. (1996). Recombinant Human Phenylalanine Hydroxylase: Novel Regulatory and Structural Properties. *Archives of Biochemistry and Biophysics*, Vol. 333, No. 1, (Sept 1996), pp.85-95, 0003-9861

Kummer, JA., Broekhuizen, R., Everett, H., Agostini, L., Kuijk, L., Martinon, F., van Bruggen, R., Tschopp, J. (2007). Inflammosome Components NALP 1 and 3 Show Distinct but Separate Expression Profiles in Human Tissues Suggesting a Site-specific Role in the Inflammatory Response. *Journal of Histochemistry & Cytochemistry*, Vol. 55, No. 5, (May 2007), pp.443-452, 0022-1554

Lacour JP., Dubois, D., Pisani, A., *et al.* (1991). Anatomical mapping of Merkel cells in normal human adult epidermis. *British Journal of Dermatology*, Vol. 125, No. 6, (Dec 1991), pp.535-542, 0007-0963

Latha, B., & Babu, M. (2001). The involvement of free radicals in burn injury: a review. *Burns*, Vol. 27, No. 4, (Jun 2001), pp.309-317, 0305-4179

Laties, AM., & Lerner, AB. (1975). Iris colour and relationship of tyrosinase activity to adrenergic innervation. *Nature*, Vol. 255, No.5504, (May 1975), pp.152-3, 0028-0836

Lazarova, R., Hristakieva, E., Lazarov, N., *et al.* (2000). Vitiligo-Related Neuropeptides in nerve Fibers of the Skin. *Archives of Physiology and Biochemistry*, Vol. 108, No. 3, (Jul 2000), pp.262-267, 1381-3455

Lepe, V., Moncada, B., Castanedo-Cazares, JP. (2003). A Double-blind Randomized Trial of 0.1% Tacrolimus vs. 0.05% Clobetasol for the Treatment of Childhood Vitiligo. *Archives of Dertmology*, Vol. 139, No. 5, (May 2003), pp. 581-585, 0003-987X

Le Poole, CI., van den Wijngaard, RMJGJ., Westerhof, W., *et al.* (1993). Presence or Absence of Melanocytes in Vitiligo Lesions: An Immunohistochemical Investigation. *Journal of Investigative Dermatology*, Vol. 100, No. 6, (Jun 1993), pp.816-822, 0022-202X

Le Poole, CI., van den Wijngaar, RMJGJ., Westerhof, W., *et al.* (1996). Presence of T cells and Macrophages in Inflammatory Vitiligo Skin Parallels Melanocyte Disappearance. *American Journal of Pathology*, Vol. 148, No. 4, (Apr 1996), pp.1219-28, 0002-9440

Le Poole, CI., van den Wijngaar, RMJGJ., Westerhof, W., *et al.* (1997). Tenascin is overexpressed in vitiligo lesional skin and inhibits melanocyte adhesion. *British Journal of Dermatology*, Vol. 137, No. 2, (Aug 1997), pp.171-178, 0007-0963

Lerner, AB. (1959). Vitiligo. *Journal of Investigative Dermatology*, Vol. 32, No. 2, (Feb 1959), pp.285-310, 0022-202X

Lewin, GR., Barde, YA. (1996). Physiology of the Neurotrophins. *Annual Reviews of Neuroscience*, Vol. 19, No. ??, (MONTH 1996), pp.289-317, 0147-006X

Li, E. (2002). Chromatin Modification and Epigenetic Reprogramming in Mammalian Development. *Nature Reviews Genetics*, Vol 3, No. 9 (Sept 2002), pp.662-73, 1471-0056

Liang, Y., Yang, S., Zhou, Y *et al.* (2007). Evidence for Two Susceptibility Loci on Chromosomes 22q12 and 6p21-p22 in Chinese Generalized Vitiligo Families. *Journal of Investigative Dermatology*, Vol. 127, No. 11, (Nov 2007), pp.2552-7, 1523-1747

Liang, C., Feng, P., Ku, B *et al.* (2006). Autophagic and tumour suppressor activity of a novel Beclin1-binding protein UVRAG. *Nature Cell Biology*, Vol. 8, No. 7, (July 2006), pp.688-91

Liu, PY., Bondesson, L., Lontz, W. (1996). The occurrence of cutaneous nerve endings and neuropeptides in vitiligo vulgaris: a case-control study. *Archives of Dermatological Research*, Vol. 288, No. 11, (Oct 1996), pp.670-675, 0340-3696

Liu, P., Pazin, DE., Merson, RR *et al.* (2008). The developmentally-regulated *Smoc2* gene is repressed by aryl-hydrocarbon receptor (Ahr) signaling. *Gene*, Vol. 433, No. 1-2, (Mar 2009), pp.72-80

Maier, S., Paulsson, M., Hartmann, U. (2008). The widely expressed extracellular matrix protein SMOC-2 promotes keratinocyte attachment and migration. *Experimental Cell Research*, Vol. 314, No. 13, (Aug 2008), pp.2477-87, 1090-2422

Majumder, PP., Das, SK., Li, CC. (1988). A Genetical Model for Vitiligo. *American Journal of Human Genetics*, Vol. 43, No. 2, (Aug 1988), pp. 119-25, 0002-9297

Manolache, L., & Benea, V. (2007). Stress in patients with alopecia areata and vitiligo. *European Academy of Dermatology and Venereology*, Vol. 21, No. 7, (Aug 2007), pp.921-928, 1468-3083

Mathews, CK., van Holde, KE., Ahern, KG. (2000). *Biochemistry*. Bejamin/Cummings, CA, USA.

Misri, R., Khopkar, U., Shankarkumar U *et al.* (2009). Comparative case control study of clinical fetures and human leukocyte antigen susceptibility between familial and nonfamilial vitiligo. *Indian Journal of Dermatology Venereology and Leprology*, Vol. 75, No. 6, (April 2009), pp.583-7

Moll, I., Bladt, U., Jung, EG. (1990). Presence of Merkel cells in sun-exposed and not sun-exposed skin: a quantitative study. *Archives of Dermatological Research*, Vol. 282, No. 4, (Oct 1990), pp.213-216

Morrone, A., Picardo, M., de Luca, C., *et al.* (1992). Catecholamines and Vitiligo. *Pigment Cell Research*, Vol. 5, No. 2, (Mar 1992), pp.65-69, 0893-5785

Nath, SK., Majumder, PP., Nordlund, JJ. (1994). Genetic epidemiology of vitiligo: multilocus recessivity cross-validated. *American Journal of Human Genetics*, Vol. 55, No. 5, (Nov 1994), pp.981-90, 0002-9297

Njoo, MD., Westerhof, W. (2001). Vitiligo: Pathogenesis and Treatment. *American Journal of Dermatology*, Vol. 2, No. 3, (MONTH 2001) pp. 167-81, 1175-0561

Nordlund, JJ. (1992). The Significance of Depigmentiation. *Pigment Cell Research Suppl*, Vol. 2 (1992), pp.237-241

Peters, EMJ., Handjiski, B., Kuhlmei, A., *et al.* (2004). Neurogenic Inflammation in Stress-Induced Termination of Murine Hair Growth is Promoted by Nerve Growth Factor. *American Journal of Pathology*, Vol. 165, No. 1, (Jul 2004), pp.259-271, 0002-9440

Philips, MA., Kingo, K., Karelson, M *et al.* (2010). Promoter polymorphism -119C/G in *MYG1* (C12orf10) gene is related to vitiligo susceptibility and Arg4Gln affects mitochondrial entrance of Myg1. *BMC Medical Genetics*, Vol. 11, No. 56, (2010), pp.1-9, 1471-2350

Prota, G. (1992). The Role of Peroxidase in Melanogenesis Revisited. *Pigment Cell Research Suppl*, Vol. 2 (1992), pp.25-31, 0893-5785

Quan, C., Ren, YQ., Xiang, LH *et al.* (2010). Genome-wide association study for vitiligo identifies susceptibility loci at 6q27 and the MHC. *Nature Genetics*, Vol. 42, No. 7, (Jul 2010), pp.614-18, 1546-1718

Rakonczay, Z., & Brimijoin, S. (1988). Biochemistry and pathophysiology of the molecular forms of cholinesterases. *Subcellular Biochemistry*, Vol. 12 (1988), 0306-0225

Rateb, AAH., Azzam, OA., Rashed, LA., *et al.* (2004). The role of nerve growth factor in the pathogenesis of vitligo. *Journal of Egyptian Women's Dermatological Society*, Vol. 1, No. 1, (2005), pp.18-24

Reik, W., Walter, J. (2001). Genomic Imprinting: Parental Influence on the Genome. *Nature Reviews Genetics*, Vol. 2, No. 1, (Jan 2001), pp.21-32, 1471-0056

Schallreuter, KU., Elwary, SMA., Gibbons, NCJ., *et al.* (2004). Activation/deactivation of acetycholinesterase by H_2O_2: more evidence for oxidative stress in vitiligo. *Biochemical and Biophysical Research Communications*, Vol. 315, No 2, (Mar 2004), pp.502-508, 0006-291X

Schallreuter, KU., Gibbons, NCJ., Zothner, C., *et al.* (2006). Butyrylcholinesterase is present int he human epidermis and is regulated by H_2O_2: more evidence for oxidative stress in vitiligo. *Biochemical and Biophysical Research Communcations*, Vol. 349, No. 3, (Oct 2006), pp.931-938, 0006-291X

Schallreuter, KU., Wood, JM., Berger, J. (1991). Low Catalase Levels in the Epidermis of Patients with Vitiligo. *Journal of Investigative Dermatology*, Vol. 87, No. 6, (Dec 1991), pp.1081-5, 0022-202X

Schallreuter, KU., Wood JM., Pittelkow, MR., *et al.* (1994). Regulation of Melanin Biosynthesis in the Human Epidermis by Tetrahydrobiopterin. *Science*, Vol. 263, No. 5152, (Mar 1994), pp.1444-1446, 0036-8075

Schreiber, SL., & Crabtree, GR. (1992). The mechanism of action of cyclosporin A and FK506. *Immunology Today*, Vol. 13, No. 4, (Apr 1992), 136-42, 0167-5699

Shalbaf, M., Gibbons, NCJ., Wood, JM., *et al.* (2008). Presence of epidermal allantoin further supports oxidative stress in vitiligo. *Experimental Dermatology*, Vol. 17, No. 9, (Sept 2008), pp.761-770, 1600-0625

Spritz, RA., Chiang, PW., Oiso, N *et al.* (2003). Human and mouse disorders of pigmentation. *Current Opinion in Genetics & Development*, Vol. 13, No. 3, (Jun 2003), pp.284-289, 0959-437X

Spritz, RA., Gowan, K., Bennett, DC., Fain, PR. (2004). Novel Vitiligo Susceptibility Loci on Chromosomes 7 (*AIS2*) and (*AIS3*), Confirmation fo *SLEV1* on Chromosome 17, and Their Roles in an Autoimmun Diathesis. *American Journal of Human Genetics*, Vol. 74, No. 1, (Jan 2004), pp. 188-191

Sravani, PV., Babu, NK., Gopal KVT., *et al.* (2009). Determination of oxidative stress in vitiligo by measuring superoxide dismutase and catalase levels in vitiliginous and non-vitiliginous skin. *Indian Journal of Dermatology Venereology and Leprology*, Vol. 75, No. 3, (May 2009), pp.268-271, 0973-3922

Stokes CE., & Sikes CR. (1988). The hypothalamic-pituitary-adrenocortical axis in major depression. *Neurologic Clinics*, Vol. 6, No. 1, (Feb 1988), pp.1-19, 0733-8619

Szalmas, A., Banati, F., Koroknai, A *et al.* (2008). Lineage-specifics silencing of human IL-10 gene expression by promoter methylation in cervical cancer cells. *European Journal of Cancer*, Vol. 44, No. 7, (May 2008), pp.1030-8, 0959-8049

Taher, ZA., Lauzon, G., Maguiness, S., *et al.* (2009). Analysis of interleukin-10 levels in lesions of vitiligo following treatment with topical tacrolimus. *British Journal of Dermatology*, Vol. 161, No. 3, (Sept 2009), pp.654-659, 1365-2133

Thompson, DM. & Parker, R. (2009). The Rnase Rny1p cleaves tRNAs and promotes cell death during oxidative stress in *Saccharomyces Cerevisiae*. *Journal of Cell Biology*, Vol. 185, No. 1, (Apr 2009), 1540-8140

Tobin, DJ., Swanson, NN., Pittelkow, MR., *et al.* (2000). Melanocytes are not absent in lesional skin of long duration of vitiligo. *Journal of Pathology*, Vol. 191, No. 4, (Aug 2000), pp.407-416, 1096-9896

Tolis G., & Stefanis, C. (1983). Depression: biological and neuroendocrine aspects. *Biomedicine and Pharmacotherapy*, Vol. 37, No. 7, (MONTH 1983), pp.316-22, 0753-3322

Tometten, M., Klapp, BF., Joachim, R., *et al.* (2004). Nerve Growth Factor and its Functional Receptor TrkA are Up-regulated in Murine Decidual Tissue of Stress-triggered and Substance P-mediated Abortion. *American Journal of Reproductive Immunology*, Vol. 51, No. 1(Jan 2004), pp.86-93, 1046-7048

Uncu, S., Yayli, S., Bahadir, S., *et al.* (2011), Relevance of autoimmune thyroiditis in children and adolescents with vitiligo. *International Journal of Dermatology*, Vol. 50, No. 2, (Feb 2011), pp.175-179, 1365-4632

Wolff, K., Johnson, RA. (2009). Section 13. Pigmentary Disorders, In: *Fitzpatrick's Color Atlas & Synopsis of Clinical Dermatology, 6e*, EDITORS, pp. Jkdf-sfjks, Publisher, Retrieved from <http://www.accessmedicine.com.login.ezproxy.library.ualberta.ca/content.aspx?aID=5187746>

Wu, CS., Yu, HS., Change, HR., *et al.* (2000). Cutaneous blood flow and adrenoceptor response increase in segmental-type vitiligo lesions. *Journal of Dermatological Science*, Vol. 23, No. 1, (May 2000), pp.53-62, 0923-1811

Yehuda, R., Brand, S., Yang, RK. (2005). Plasma Neuropeptide Y Concentrations in Combat Exposed Veterans: Relationship to Trauma Exposure, Recovery from PTSD, and Coping. *Biological Psychiatry*, Vol. 59, No. 7, (Apr 2006), pp.660-663, 0006-3223

Yildirim, M., Baysal, V., Inaloz, HS., *et al.* (2004). The role of oxidants and antioxidants in generalized vitiligo at tissue level. *Journal of European Academy of Dermatology and Venereology*, Vol. 18, No. 6, (Nov 2004), pp.683-686, 0926-9959

Yoshimura, T., Matsuyama, W., Kamohara, H. (2005). Discoidin Domain Receptor 1: *A New Class of Receptor Regulating Leukocyte-Collagen Interaction. Immunologic Research*, Vol. 31, No. 3, (2005), pp.219-229, 0257-277X

Yun, JY., Uhm, YK., Kim, HJ *et al.* (2010). Tranforming growth factor beta receptor II (TGFBR2) polymorphisms and the association with nonsegmental vitiligo inthe Korean population. *International Journal of Immunogenetics*, Vol. 37, No. 4, (Aug 2010), pp.289-91

Zhao, M., Gao, F., Wu, J *et al.* (2010). Abnormal DNA methylation in peripheral blood mononuclear cells from patients with vitiligo. *British Journal of Dermatology*, Vol. 163, No. 4, (Oct 2010), pp.736-742, 1365-2133

3

The Psychosocial Aspects of Vitiligo: A Focus on Stress Involvement in Children with Vitiligo

Liana Manolache
Cetatea Histria Polyclinic, Bucharest
Romania

1. Introduction

Skin interacts with the environment and serves as a means to communicate. Skin diseases can affect both self-image and social relationships, particularly during the vulnerable times of childhood and adolescence. Vitiligo itself has more than a 3000 year history, with the first reports of the condition chronicled in early Vedic and Egyptian texts; vitiligo was often confused with leprosy and led to greater stigmatization of affected individuals (Millington and Levell, 2007).

The psychosocial aspects of vitiligo can be described by stress as a potential cause or effect of the disease, the anxiety or depression of vitiligo patients, or the impact of vitiligo on patient quality of life.

There are few reports of the psychosocial impact of vitiligo on children and adolescents although vitiligo can have a serious impact on their lives. This ranges from vitiligo having no correlation with stress (Prcic *et al.*, 2006) to involvement of stressful events in 50% of cases (Barisic-Drusko & Rucevic, 2004). Psychological vulnerability can also influence the onset and evolution of psychosomatic dermatoses, alongside the presence of stressful events. A recent study (Schwartz *et al.*, 2009) on the temperament of children with vitiligo revealed that these children score high on the "harm avoidance" scale, meaning that compared to their healthy siblings, children with vitiligo seem to have a greater fear of strangers and have a heightened response to any changes in a close relative. Age, change of location, and situational or environmental alterations can also be predictors of stress.

About half of vitiligo vulgaris patients have onset of their illness during childhood, which can increase psychological distress during the formative years (Siverberg, 2010). On the other hand, in the prepubertal period, children are not focused yet on their physical appearance, so an early onset could also act as a "protective factor", enabling the child to develop compensatory mechanisms of coping with disease and ways to strengthen self-esteem (Hill-Boeuf & Porter, 1984).

We performed a pivotal study to add to this body of knowledge, with the purpose of observing stress involvement before the onset of childhood vitiligo and during its subsequent progression. Furthermore, we relate this to the psychosocial aspects of all vitiligo patients, making our study relevant to the disease entity as a whole.

2. A pivotal study of stress involvement in children with vitiligo

Our study was performed at the Department of Dermatology of Cetatea Histria Polyclinic in Bucharest, Romania. Patients (children and adults) were referred to the polyclinic by general practitioners in the city and its surrounding areas (approximately 500,000 inhabitants). There were 41 cases of vitiligo in 9,940 new dermatology consults in children less than 16 years of age from the time period between March 2001 and December 2007. The incidence of vitiligo was 0.45% of all dermatologic conditions in children.
Nearly 83% (34/41) of childhood vitiligo cases had disease onset less than 9 months before evaluation or had recent progression and these cases were included in our analysis. The study design was case-control, with each patient having an age- and gender-matched counterpart. Controls had skin diseases with a well-established etiology with a presumably low psychosomatic component, or had skin diseases unrelated to stress (*e.g.*bacterial, viral, and fungal infections, Table 1). We selected interviews with children and parents taking into consideration potential stressful situations that appeared during the year before evaluation and excluding those that occurred after onset or exacerbation of disease. This was based on the theory that life events can influence susceptibility to vitiligo through increased levels of stress.
The situations reported were classified into: events related to school and education, family changes, personal illnesses/accidents/surgeries, and psychosocial trauma (frightening situations to children). This classification, made after the collection of data, could be considered arbitrary without other references, but we determined this categorization to underline the importance of events related to events of importance in childhood.
Odds ratios were calculated and χ^2 and t tests were used in order to study the differences between the groups, and used the standard significance value of $p \leq 0.05$.

2.1 Results

2.1.1 Demographics

There were 16 girls (47%) and 18 boys (53%) in the vitiligo group. Mean age was 11 years old (standard deviation, SD=3.1). There was no significant difference (p=0.38) between the mean age in girls (10.5 years- SD=3.18) and boys (11.44 years, SD=3.05).
Most of children (38%) had recent onset (less than 3 months) of disease or recent progression (an additional 38%). The youngest child with vitiligo was 4 years old. Nearly 21% of children had a family history of vitiligo. One in five children had divorced parents. Halo nevi were observed in 15% of patients. Associated thyroid dysfunction was found in 1 girl and 1 boy (6%). Boys had mostly acrofacial lesions and girls most commonly had vitiligo vulgaris.
Data regarding mean age, distribution according to age group, lesion type, family, and onset of lesions was collected (Table 1).

2.1.2 Stress involvement

In vitiligo group, 18 o f 34 (53%) children mentioned a stressful event compared to 6 of the controls (17.6%). The difference was statistically significant (χ^2 =7.79, p=0.005). The odds ratio was 5.25 [95% CI: 1.73-15.92]. Girls experienced mostly one event with an important impact on vitiligo, compared to boys who reported between 1-3 related events. In the vitiligo group, girls with acrofacial lesions and boys with vitiligo vulgaris were most often affected by stressful situations. These were situations related to school (beginning of education, exams, over-solicitation, or change of school). Psychosocial trauma was also a key impact factor (Tables 2-4).

	Females	Males	Total (%)
Family			
Only child	7	8	-
Socio-professional level			
High	5	6	32
Average	6	9	44
Low*	5	2	23.5
Separated/divorced parents	2	5	20.6
Onset of Lesions			
< 3 months	7	6	38
3-6 months	2	4	
6-9 months	0	2	
Recent progression	7	6	38
Vitiligo Type			
Acro-facial	4	10	41
Vulgaris	3	4	20.6
Focal	9	4	38.2
Mean Age	10.5 years (SD=3.18)	11.44 years (SD=3.05)	11 years (SD=3.1)
Age			
1. <5 years	1	0	
2. 5-9 years old	7	6	38.2
3. 10-14 years old	8	12	58.8
Controls			
Mycosis	1	2	
Tinea pedis	0	0	
Tinea manuum	2	3	
Tinea corporis/faciei	5	7	
Pityriasis versicolor	5	2	
Verruca	3	4	
Impetigo			

*mother housewife or one parent unemployed/retired

Table 1. Demographic Data

Number of events	Vitiligo Group (n=34)				Control Group (n=34)				(p)*		
	Females	Males	Total		Females		Males	Total	Fem.	Mal.	Total
	Mean/ SD	Mean/ SD	Mean	SD	Mean /SD	Mean /SD	Mean	SD			
	0.625/ 0.61	0.83/ 1.04	**0.73**	0.86	0.18/ 0.39	0.16/ 0.37	**0.17**	0.38	0.01	**0.01**	**0.009**
	N	**N**	**N**	%	**N**	**N**	**N**	%			
1 event	8	5	**13**		3	3	**6**				
2 events	1	2	**3**	72.2	0	0	**0**	100%			
3 events	0	2	**2**								

*SD= standard deviation
N= number of cases

Table 2. Comparison of Stressful Events in Vitiligo

	Vitiligo Vulgaris	Acro-Facial Vitiligo	Focal Vitiligo
Females			
- Number of cases	9	4	3
- History of stress	4	3	2
Males			
- Number of cases	4	10	4
- History of stress	3	5	1

Table 3. Comparison of Stress Involvement

Type of event	Vitiligo group			Control group			(p)		
	Females	Males	Total	Females	Males	Total	Females	Males	Total
1. ***Related to School and Education***	4	3	7	3	3	6	0.6	0.6	0.49
- Beginning of school	3	1	4	2	0	2			
- Examinations	0	1	1	1	1	2			
- Change of school or class	0	1	1	0	0	0			
- Problems/too many homeworks or studies	1	0	1	0	2	2			

Type of event	Vitiligo group			Control group			(p)		
	Females	Males	Total	Females	Males	Total	Females	Males	Total
2. ***Familial Issues***	1	3	4						
- disputes	1	0	1						
- death of a family member	0	1	1						
- change of residence	0	1	1						
- new person in the family	0	1	1						
3. ***Personal Events***									
-illness/accident/ operation	1	1	2						
4. ***Psychosocial Trauma***	0	1	1						

Table 4. Types of Stressful Events in Vitiligo and Control Patients

3. Discussion

The spectrum of incidence for vitiligo in the pediatric population ranges from 0.09% in Singapore (Giam, 1998) and Denmark (Howitz et al., 1977) to 2.6% in India (Jaisankar et al., 1992), 4.1% in Thailand (Wisuthsarewong & Viravan, 2000) and 5% in Eastern Saudi Arabia (Alakloby, 2005). Studies that reported vitiligo is more common in females: India (Handa &Dogra, 2003, Jaisankar et al., 1992), Kuwait (Nanda et al., 1999), Croatia (Prcic et al., 2006), China (Lin et al, 2011), differed from our data. The mean age (11 years old) of our cohort was higher than other reports (between 6.2 years to 9 years) (Handa & Dogra, 2003, Hu et al., 2006, Nanda et al., 1999, Prcic et al., 2006). A family history of vitiligo (about 20%) was comparable to those of Akrem's (18%) (Akrem et al., 2008), but higher than of Lin's (Lin et al., 2011) (13.5%). There are other results from 12-13% (Cho et al., 2000, Handa & Dogra, 2003) up to 27% (Al-Mutairi et al., 2005). The dimensions of our study sample could be considered a limitation and account for differences in demographics from other studies.

3.1 Stress involvement

There is a lack of studies in pediatric dermatology to which to compare our data. Our results, which found that 53% of pediatric patients reported stress involvement in the natural history of their disease, was statistically significant: $\chi^2 = 7.79$, p=0.005 with an odds ratio of 5.25. The percentage of stress involvement seems to be consistent with the results of Barisic-Drusko[3] and their study of childhood vitiligo compared to childhood psoriasis mentioned that in children with vitiligo (n=65), onset was related to psychological factors in 56.9% of cases compared to children with psoriasis, in which onset was mostly related to the presence of an inflammatory focus. Stress seemed to appear more often in segmental vitiligo[14]. However, there are also reports that did not find a significant correlation of childhood vitiligo with the presence of stressful events (Prcic et al., 2006).

Based on this data, periods of adjustment to new conditions, such as the beginning of education (school or kindergarten), being an only child, or having separated parents (particularly in boys) could be considered special situations in which children with vitiligo need more support and require the intervention of families, teachers and doctors.

In a previous study with a smaller sample size, we found an even higher rate of stress involvement (57%) (Manolache et al., 2009a) in children with vitiligo. We also studied, in a similarly designed case-control study, children with alopecia areata (43 cases) and psoriasis (41 cases). In the alopecia areata group, we found stress involvement in 58% of cases (16% in controls). This difference was strongly significant (χ^2 =14.36, $p<0.0001$). The odds ratio was 7.14 [95% CI: 2.59-19.63]. There was no difference between girls (60%) and boys (55.5%) (Manolache et al., 2009b). The types of events reported by children with alopecia areata were mostly related to school, *i.e.,* beginning school or kindergarten, exams, change of class or school, problems with schoolmates or teachers, too many classes or homework, children feeling over-solicited (56%). In children with psoriasis, stress was present in 41% of cases. Girls with psoriasis vulgaris and boys with guttate lesions were more often affected by stressful situations. Family issues (death, illnesses, disputes, parents working abroad, financial restrictions) were more often described, but school- related problems (exams or beginning school) were also prevalent.

In regards to adults, the importance of stressful events and the number of these events before the onset of vitiligo has been described in several case-control studies (Manolache &Benea, 2007, Papadopoulos et al., 1998). Stress is cited in 62-65% of patients (Firooz et al., 2004, Manolache & Benea 2007). Patients with vitiligo had a significant number of stressful events in the year preceding the onset of the disease as compared to controls (Prcic et al., 2006). In Agarwal's study (Agarwal, 1998), half of the patients with vitiligo reported stressful events before disease onset. Meanwhile, other reports (Picardi et al., 2003) found no differences between vitiligo patients and controls when comparing numbers of stressful events.

In our previous study, we found significant differences in the mean number of stressful events only between women with vitiligo and controls. There was no difference with men or the vitiligo cohort as a whole. These results were concordant with respect to those of Picardi *et al.*(Picardi et al., 2003). They also found no differences between vitiligo patients and controls regarding the total number of stressful events or the number of undesirable, uncontrollable, or major events. The difference between patients and controls was related to exposure to three or more uncontrollable events, which were more often reported by vitiligo patients. They suggest that alexthymia (the inability to verbally express emotions), insecure attachments, and poor social support systems could reduce patients' ability to cope with stress and could increase susceptibility to vitiligo.

Potential stressful situations reported in other vitiligo studies were marital or financial problems (Papadopoulos et al., 1998), loss of loved ones (*e.g.,* death, separation), illnesses, and changes in eating or sleeping habits (Papadopoulos et al., 1998). In a study by Silvan (Silvan, 2004), 40% of vitiligo patients experienced the death of a close friend or family member. In comparison, 25% of vitiligo patients experienced loss in a study by Papadopoulos; loss in this case meaning relocation, or the loss of friends, family, or familiar surroundings (Papadopoulos et al., 1998, Silvan, 2004).

Patients with vitiligo often have different perceptions of the etiology of their disease. Often, they believe that stress (30-60% of cases) or genetic background (24-32% of cases) may play a role (AlGhamdi, 2010, Firooz et al., 2004).

3.2 Psychiatric symptomology

Vitiligo patients tend to have high scores for anxiety (Gieler et al., 2000, Mechri et al., 2006), depression (Agarwal, 1998, Mechri et al., 2006), adjustment disorders (Mattoo et al., 2002), obsessive symptoms, and hypochondriasis (Elgowieni et al., 2003). Furthermore, depressive illnesses, generalized anxiety, mixed anxiety and depression, social phobia, agoraphobia, and sexual dysfunction are also common in vitiligo patients(Mechri et al., 2006). Patients with vitiligo also have high rates of alexthymia and avoidant behaviors (Picardi et al., 2003).

There are some studies comparing vitiligo (113 cases) with psoriasis (103 cases) that have found psychiatric morbidity in 33.63% of vitiligo patients compared to 24 7% of psoriasis patients (Mattoo et al., 2001). Sharma (Sharma et al., 2001) also made a comparison between psoriasis and vitiligo patients. They found depression in 23.3% of psoriasis patients and in 10% of vitiligo patients. Anxiety was found in equal rates in both groups (3.3%). Sleep disturbances were a problem in 56.6% of psoriasis patients and in 20% of vitiligo patients.

There are few studies on children with vitiligo and psychiatric symptomology. One study showed children with vitiligo were more depressed than non-affected children (Bilgic et al., 2010). Another study found no differences between children and adolescents with vitiligo and healthy subjects in regards to anxiety and depression (Prcic et al., 2006).

Vitiligo patients who cope well with their condition have higher self-esteem than individuals without the disorder. Those who cope poorly have significantly lower self-esteem, which suggests that response to disfiguring diseases is affected by basic ego strength. Younger patients and those individuals in lower socioeconomic groups show particularly poor adjustment skills (Porter et al., 1979).

3.3 Quality of life

Vitiligo has a definite psychosocial impact in adolescents that is correlated with lesion severity . The duration of the illness is directly related to physical health score (meaning physical functioning on the Pediatric Quality of Life Inventory [PedsQoL]) in children. Involvement of the face, head, or neck in boys and involvement of the genital area and legs in girls were related to impaired quality of life. Disease location may be considered important because of its effects on gender identity development (Bilgic et al., 2010).

Patients reporting negative childhood experiences described significantly more problems in social development than those who did not report negative experiences. Negative childhood experiences were significantly associated with more health- related quality of life (HRQoL, a self-reported measure of physical and mental health) impairments in early adulthood (Linthorst et al., 2008). The quality of life of adolescents with vitiligo is closely related to patient apprehension of the disease, ability to make psychosocial adjustments, and presence of psychiatric comorbidity, rather than the clinical severity of the condition itself (Choi et al., 2009). Age plays an extremely important part in adjustment to disease, with the junior high school years (11 to 14 years old) being particularly traumatic. Change of location or situation is a predictor of vitiligo-related stress. It is important to note, however, that children who develop other competencies that build self-esteem cope better with vitiligo (Hill-Boeuf & Porter, 1984).

More than half of vitiligo patients (56.5%) indicated that vitiligo moderately or severely affects their quality of life (Talsania et al., 2010). Dermatology Life Quality Index (DLQI) is the first dermatology-specific quality of life questionnaire developed in 1994, composed of 10 simple questions validated in different languages. The scores range from 0 to 30 (0-1: no effect on patient's life, 2-5: small effect, 6-10: moderate effect, 11-20: very large effect, 21-30: extremely large effect). The score in most studies represents a moderate impact of vitiligo on quality of life (6-10) (Dolatshahi et al., 2008, Kostopoulou et al., 2009, Mechri et al., 2006, Ongenae et al., 2005a, Radtke et al., 2009). The highest mean DLQI value was observed in the patient group aged 20-29 years (Radtke et al., 2009). Perceived severity and patient's personality were predictors of quality of life impairment (Kostopoulou et al., 2009). There were statistically significant relationships between DLQI scores and marital status, skin phototype, and disease progression, respectively (Al Robaee, 2007, Dolatshahi et al., 2008, Ongenae et al., 2005a). In particular, there was found to be a connection between impaired health-related quality of life and unstable marital relationships (Wang et al., 2011). Furthermore, vitiligo also negatively impacts the sexual lives of patients (Sukan &Maner, 2007).

Vitiligo of the face, head, and neck regions substantially affects DLQI, independently of the degree of disease involvement (Ongenae et al., 2005a). Quality of life is significantly impaired in females to a greater extent than males, as well as in cases affecting more than 10% of the body surface area (Belhadjali et al., 2007). Al Robaee (Al Robaee, 2007) observed that women are more embarrassed and self-conscious about their disease than men, as it impairs social life, personal relationships, sexual activities, and choice of clothing. The same study (Al Robaee, 2007), revealed a great impact of vitiligo on patients (DLQI 14.72). A significant correlation was noted between quality of life scores and depression as well as anxiety scores, respectively (Mechri et al., 2006).

DLQI scores do tend to be lower for vitiligo patients than for psoriasis patients (Ongenae et al., 2005b, Radtke et al., 2009), as vitiligo patients seem to exhibit better adjustment to their disease and experience less social discrimination than do psoriasis patients, however, the two groups do not differ on overall self-esteem scores (Porter et al., 1986).

Studies using Skindex-29 (SD-29, a dermatologic HRQoL instrument) to evaluate the quality of life revealed that patients with vitiligo were highly affected in both the functional and emotional aspects of QOL, with some sex differences (Kim et al., 2009). Generalized vitiligo, darker skin types, vitiligo located on the chest, and treatment in the past appeared to have an adverse impact on the psychosocial domains of quality of life (Linthorst et al., 2009).

3.4 Stigmatization

Stigmatization also plays an important part in the lives of vitiligo patients (Ongenae et al., 2005a). Avoidance and concealment of the disease are commonplace. Experiences of stigmatization are often perceived to be associated with cultural values related to appearance, status, and myths linked to the cause of the condition (Thompson et al., 2010). Patients with visible lesions are more prone to stigmatization (Schmid-Ott et al., 2007). Self-esteem and perceived stigmatization are significantly associated with degree of disturbance to the patient. Gender, age, and visibility of the condition are not significantly related to degree of disturbance, although an indirect relationship is observed.

4. Conclusion

Stressful situations can be correlated with the onset or progression of vitiligo. Often, one stressful situation with an important impact on a child's emotional balance is sufficient enough to trigger or exacerbate disease. Periods of adjustment to new conditions such as beginning education and school, being an only child, or having separated parents are reported to be important in terms of psychosocial impact for children with vitiligo and may require intervention.

In general, it is important to take into consideration the entire psychosocial profile of vitiligo patients, in particular pediatric patients. These are key to identifying potential stress-related triggers, predicting type of patient personality or psychological reactions due to vitiligo, and evaluating the impact of disease on patient quality of life.

5. References

Agarwal G. (1998) Vitiligo: an under-estimated problem. *Fam Pract* 1998; 15 (Suppl. 1): S19–S23.

Akrem J, Baroudi A, Aichi T, Houch F, Hamdaoui MH. (2008) Profile of vitiligo in the south of Tunisia. *Int J Dermatol.* 2008 Jul;47(7):670-4

Alakloby OM. (2005) Pattern of skin diseases in Eastern Saudi Arabia. *Saudi Med J.* 2005 Oct;26(10):1607-10.

AlGhamdi KM. (2010) Beliefs and perceptions of Arab vitiligo patients regarding their condition. *Int J Dermatol.* 2010 Oct;49(10):1141-5.

Al-Mutairi N, Sharma AK, Al-Sheltawy M,Nour-Eldin O. (2005) Childhood vitiligo: a prospective hospital-based study. *Australas J Dermatol.* 2005 Aug;46(3):150-3.

Al Robaee AA. (2007) Assessment of quality of life in Saudi patients with vitiligo in a medical school in Qassim province, Saudi Arabia. *Saudi Med J.* 2007 Sep;28(9):1414-7.

Barisic-Drusko V, Rucevic I (2004) Trigger factors in childhood psoriasis and vitiligo. *Coll Antropol* 2004; 28(1): 277-85.

Belhadjali H, Amri M, Mecheri A, Doarika A, Khorchani H, Youssef M, Gaha L, Zili J. (2007) [Vitiligo and quality of life: a case-control study]. *Ann Dermatol Venereol.* 2007 Mar;134(3 Pt 1):233-6.

Bilgic O, Bilgic A, Akis HK, Eskioglu F, Kilic EZ. (2011) Depression, anxiety and health-related quality of life in children and adolescents with vitiligo. *Clin Exp Dermatol.* 2011 Jun;36(4):360-5. doi: 10.1111/j.1365-2230.2010.03965.x. Epub 2010 Dec 24.

Cho S, Kang HC, Hahm JH. (2000) Characteristics of vitiligo in Korean children. *Pediatr Dermatol.* 2000 May-Jun;17(3):189-93.

Choi S, Kim DY, Whang SH, Lee JH, Hann SK, Shin YJ. (2010) Quality of life and psychological adaptation of Korean adolescents with vitiligo. *J Eur Acad Dermatol Venereol.* 2010 May;24(5):524-9. Epub 2009 Oct 6.

Dolatshahi M, Ghazi P, Feizy V, Hemami MR. (2008) Life quality assessment among patients with vitiligo: comparison of married and single patients in Iran. *Indian J Dermatol Venereol Leprol.* 2008 Nov-Dec;74(6):700.

Elgowieni M, Ramadan I, Molukia T.(2003) Vitiligo: its personality profile. *Dermatol Psychosom* 2003; 4: 107.

Firooz A, Bouzari N, Fallah N et al. (2004) What patients with vitiligo think about their condition. *Int J Dermatol* 2004; 43: 811–814.

Giam YC. (1998) Skin diseases in children in Singapore. *Ann Acad Med Singapore.* 1998 Oct;17(4):569-72

Gieler U, Brosig B, Schneider U et al.(2000) Vitiligo-coping behavior. *Dermatol Psychosom* 2000; 1: 6–10.

Handa S, Dogra S. (2003) Epidemiology of childhood vitiligo: a study of 625 patients from north India. *Pediatr Dermatol.* 2003 May-Ju;20(3):207-10

Hill-Boeuf A, Porter JD. (1984) Children coping with impaired appearance: social and psychological influences. *Gen Hosp Psychiatry* 1984 Oct;6(4):294-301

Howitz J, Brodhagen H, Schwartz M, Thomsen K. (1977) Prevalence of vitiligo. Epidemiological survey on the Isle of Bornholm, Denmark.*Arch Dermatol.* 1977 Jan;113(1):47-52

Hu Z, Liu JB, Ma SS, Yang S, Zhang XJ. (2006) Profile of childhood vitiligo in China: an analysis of 541 patients. *Pediatr Dermatol.* 2006 Mar-Apr;23(2):114-6.

Jaisankar TJ, Baruah MC, Garg BR. (1992) Vitiligo in children. *Int J Dermatol.* 1992 Sep;31(9):621-3

Kim do Y, Lee JW, Whang SH, Park YK, Hann SK, Shin YJ. (2009) Quality of life for Korean patients with vitiligo: Skindex-29 and its correlation with clinical profiles. *J Dermatol.* 2009 Jun;36(6):317-22. Epub 2009 Apr 28.

Kostopoulou P, Jouary T, Quintard B, Ezzedine K, Marques S, Boutchnei S, Taieb A.(2009) Objective vs. subjective factors in the psychological impact of vitiligo: the experience from a French referral centre. *Br J Dermatol.* 2009 Jul;161(1):128-33. Epub 2009 Mar 9.

Lin X, Tang LY, Fu WW, Kang KF (2011) Childhood vitiligo in China: clinical profiles and immunological findings in 620 cases. *Am J Clin Dermatol.* 2011 Aug 1;12(4):277-81. doi: 10.2165/11318020-000000000-00000.

Linthorst Homan MW, de Korte J, Grootenhuis MA, Bos JD, Sprangers MA, van der Veen JP. (2008) Impact of childhood vitiligo on adult life. *Br J Dermatol.* 2008 Sep;159(4):915-20. Epub 2008 Aug 20.

Linthorst Homan MW, Spuls PI, de Korte J, Bos JD, Sprangers MA, van der Veen JP (2009) The burden of vitiligo: patient characteristics associated with quality of life. *J Am Acad Dermatol.* 2009 Sep;61(3):411-20. Epub 2009 Jul 3.

Manolache L, Benea V. (2007) Stress in patients with alopecia areata and vitiligo *J Eur Acad Dermatol Venereol* 2007, 21, 921–928

Manolache L, Petrescu-Seceleanu D, Benea V (2009a). Correlation of stressful events with onset of vitiligo in children. *J Eur Acad Dermatol Venereol.* 2009,23, 187-88.

Manolache L, Petrescu-Seceleanu D, Benea V (2009b). Alopecia areata and relationship with stressful events in children. *J Eur Acad Dermatol Venereol.* 2009,23, 107-8.

Mattoo SK, Handa S, Kaur I, Gupta N, Malhotra R. (2001) Psychiatric morbidity in vitiligo and psoriasis: a comparative study from India. *J Dermatol* 2001; 28: 424–432.

Mattoo SK, Handa S, Kaur I, Gupta N, Malhotra R. (2002) Psychiatric morbidity in vitiligo: prevalence and correlates in India. *J Eur Acad Dermatol Venereol* 2002; 16: 573–578.

Mechri A, Amri M, Douarika AA, Ali Hichem BH, Zouari B, Zili J.(2006) [Psychiatric morbidity and quality of life in Vitiligo: a case controlled study]. *Tunis Med.* 2006 Oct;84(10):632-5.

Millington GW, Levell NJ. Vitiligo: the historical curse of depigmentation. *Int J Dermatol.* 2007 Sep;46(9):990-5.

Nanda A, Al-Hasawi F, Alsaleh QA. (1999) A prospective survey of pediatric dermatology clinic patients in Kuwait: an analysis of 10,000 cases. *Pediatr Dermatol.*1999 Jan-Feb;16(1):6-11

Ongenae K, Van Geel N, De Schepper S, Naeyaert JM. (2005) Effect of vitiligo on self-reported health-related quality of life.*Br J Dermatol.* 2005 Jun;152(6):1165-72.

Ongenae K, Dierckxsens L, Brochez L, van Geel N, Naeyaert JM. (2006) Quality of life and stigmatization profile in a cohort of vitiligo patients and effect of the use of camouflage. *Dermatology.* 2005;210(4):279-85.

Papadopoulos L, Bor R, Legg C, Hawk JL.(1998) Impact of life events on the onset of vitiligo in adults: preliminary evidence for a psychological dimension in aetiology. *Clin Exp Dermatol* 1998; 23: 243–248.

Prcic S, Durovic D, Duran V, Vukovic D, Gajinov Z. (2006) Some psychological characteristics of children and adolescents with vitiligo--our results. *Med Pregl.* 2006 May-Jun;59(5-6):265-9.

Picardi A, Pasquini P, Cattaruzza MS et al. (2003) Stressful life events, social support, attachment security and alexithymia in vitiligo. A case-control study. *Psychother Psychosom* 2003; 72: 150–158.

Porter JR, Beuf AH, Lerner A, Nordlund J. (1986) Psychosocial effect of vitiligo: a comparison of vitiligo patients with "normal" control subjects, with psoriasis patients, and with patients with other pigmentary disorders. *J Am Acad Dermatol.* 1986 Aug;15(2 Pt 1):220-4.

Porter J, Beuf AH, Nordlund JJ, Lerner AB. (1979)Psychological reaction to chronic skin disorders: a study of patients with vitiligo. *Gen Hosp Psychiatry.* 1979 Apr;1(1):73-7.

Radtke MA, SchÃ¤fer I, Gajur A, Langenbruch A, Augustin M. (2009) Willingness-to-pay and quality of life in patients with vitiligo. *Br J Dermatol.* 2009 Jul;161(1):134-9. Epub 2009 Mar 9.

Schmid-Ott G, Kansebeck HW, Jecht E, Shimshoni R, Lazaroff I, Schallmayer S, Calliess IT, Malewski P, Lamprecht F, Gatz A. (2007) Stigmatization experience, coping and sense of coherence in vitiligo patients. *J Eur Acad Dermatol Venereol.* 2007 Apr;21(4):456-61.

Schwartz R, Sepulveda JE, Quintana T. (2009) Possible role of psychological and environmental factors in the genesis of childhood vitiligo. *Rev Med Chil,* 2009 Jan;137(1):53-62.

Sharma N, Koranne RV, Singh RK. (2001) Psychiatric morbidity in psoriasis and vitiligo: a comparative study. *J Dermatol* 2001; 28: 419–423.

Silvan M. (2004) The psychological aspects in vitiligo. *Cutis* 2004; 73: 163–167.

Siverberg NB. (2010) Update on childhood vitiligo. *Curr Opin Pediatr,* 2010 Aug:22(4):445-52

Sukan M, Maner F. (2007) The problems in sexual functions of vitiligo and chronic urticaria patients. *J Sex Marital Ther.* 2007 Jan-Feb;33(1):55-64.

Talsania N, Lamb B, Bewley A.(2010) Vitiligo is more than skin deep: a survey of members of the Vitiligo Society. *Clin Exp Dermatol.* 2010 Oct;35(7):736-9. doi: 10.1111/j.1365-2230.2009.03765.x.

Thompson AR, Clarke SA, Newell RJ, Gawkrodger DJ (2010) Appearance Research Collaboration (ARC) Vitiligo linked to stigmatization in British South Asian women: a qualitative study of the experiences of living with vitiligo. *Br J Dermatol.* 2010 Sep;163(3):481-6. doi: 10.1111/j.1365-2133.2010.09828.x. Epub 2010 Apr 26.

Wang KY, Wang KH, Zhang ZP. (2011) Health-related quality of life and marital quality of vitiligo patients in China. *J Eur Acad Dermatol Venereol.* 2011 Apr;25(4):429-35. doi: 10.1111/j.1468-3083.2010.03808.x.

Wisuthsarewong W, Viravan S. (2000) Analysis of skin diseases in a referral pediatric dermatology clinic in Thailand. *J Med Assoc Thai.* 2000 Sep;83(9):999-1004

Ultraviolet B (UVB) Phototherapy in the Treatment of Vitiligo

Kelly KyungHwa Park[1] and Jenny Eileen Murase[1,2]
[1]University of California San Francisco
Department of Dermatology, San Francisco, California
[2]Palo Alto Foundation Medical Group
Department of Dermatology, Mountain View, California
USA

1. Introduction

Vitiligo is a common, acquired pigmentary disorder of unknown pathogenesis that presents a therapeutic challenge to many dermatologists (Figure 1). Although surgery in the form of grafting or transplantation is generally the most definitive treatment option, these procedures are limited by concerns of post-procedure cosmesis. Photochemotherapy using psoralen and ultraviolet A (PUVA) therapy, topical and oral immunosuppresants, as well as cosmetic camouflage are also commonly employed with varying clinical efficacy. Phototherapy is a popular treatment option, which includes both of the generalized ultraviolet B (UVB) therapies, broadband UVB (BB-UVB) and narrowband UVB (NB-UVB). The UVB-based therapeutic modalities in development are targeted delivery of BB- and NB-UVB, monochromatic excimer light (MEL), microphototherapy, and combination therapy. In particular, the sophisticated devices that utilize MEL can emit coherent 308-nm radiation using the xenon chloride (XeCl) excimer laser or microphotography, while incoherent radiation can be supplied by various lamp and light systems. All of the UVB phototherapy modalities can be used in combination with topical or systemic agents, thus further expanding treatment options for vitiligo patients.

2. History

The use of ultraviolet (UV) irradiation was introduced into the field of dermatology in the 1800s after its Nobel Prize-winning application in lupus vulgaris (Roelandts, 2002). By 1928, UV radiation was used in the Goeckerman regimen as part of the classic crude coal tar and phototherapy treatment for psoriasis. Decades later in 1978, BB-UVB phototherapy was developed and used for psoriasis and pruritus. NB-UVB originated in Europe in 1988 indicated for psoriasis, and soon became widely used in the United States in the 1990s. Its innovative use in vitiligo came nearly a decade later in 1997 (Wiskemann 1978; Westerhof and Nieuweboer-Krobotova, 1997). The pivotal study introducing NB-UVB use in vitiligo demonstrated that more patients undergoing NB-UVB had repigmentation of vitiligo patches than those who underwent PUVA photochemotherapy (67% vs. 46%) (Westerhof and Nieuweboer-Krobotova, 1997). Since then, the use of UVB for vitiligo has become commonplace, and new technologic developments in UVB therapy are continuously underway. The use of MEL with the excimer laser was first described in 1997 (Bonis, Kemeny et al., 1997).

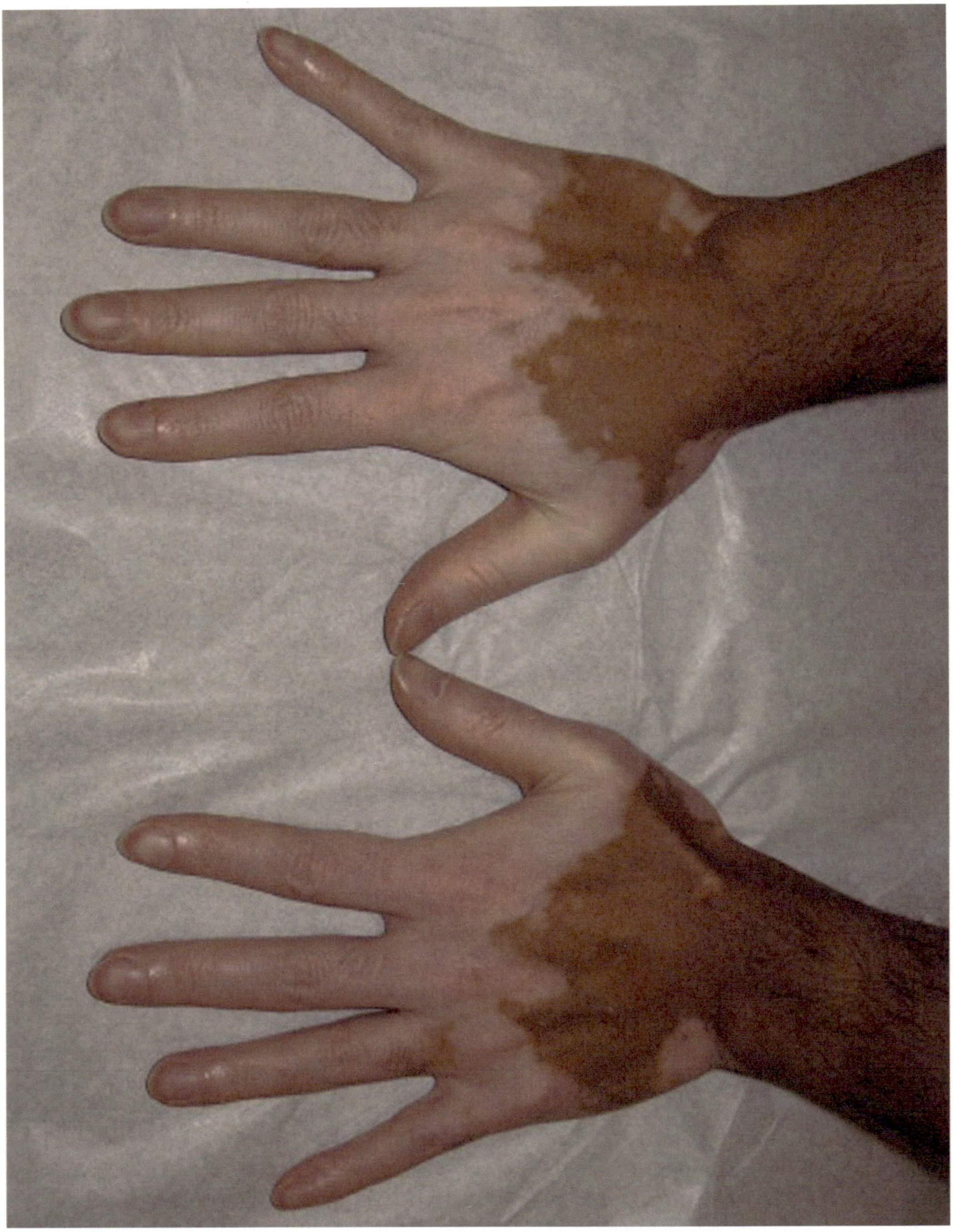

Fig. 1. Vitiligo of the hands.

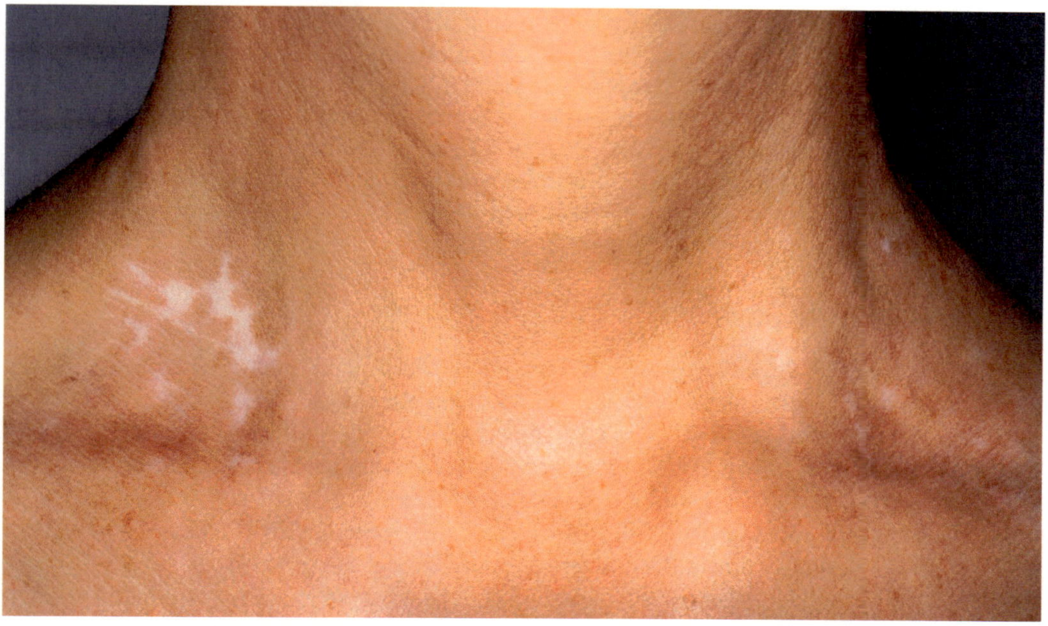

Fig. 2. Near complete repigmention of vitiligo patches with NB-UVB treatment.

3. Theory and mechanism of action

UVB phototherapy consists of the use of artificial light without the use of adjunct photosensitizing agents. It is used for a variety of dermatological conditions, including psoriasis, atopic dermatitis and other eczematous disorders, pruritus, graft-versus-host-disease, lichen planus, and seborrheic dermatitis, among others. In vitiligo, UVB phototherapy ideally results in repigmentation, disease control, and prevention of progression of vitiligo through its immunosuppressive and immunomodulatory properties. UVB is available for use in vitiligo as BB-UVB (290-320 nanometers, nm), NB-UVB (310-312 nm), and monochromatic excimer light (MEL, 308 nm). Although the action spectrum or wavelength(s) specifically targeting vitiligo has yet to be determined, both BB- and NB-UVB as well as MEL have been demonstrated to be clinically effective.

The mechanism of how UVB works in vitiligo is unknown. It is established that distinct UVB radiation wavelengths target particular chromophores in the skin, in particular keratinocytes and melanocytes in the epidermis and fibroblasts in the dermis, and facilitate the therapeutic mechanisms of the light depending on chromophore type and function. In the case of UVB, these include apoptosis induction, T-cell depletion, decreased antigen presentation, and the ability to regulate inflammatory mediators and cytokines (Novak, Bonis et al., 2002; Novak, Berces et al., 2004; Weichenthal and Schwarz, 2005).

UV, in particular, NB-UVB, is presumed to stimulate dopa-lacking amelanotic melanocytes in the outer root sheaths of hair follicles to produce melanin (Cui, Shen et al., 1991; Norris, Horikawa et al., 1994). It also activates melanocyte migration to adjacent depigmented areas, causing perifollicular repigmentation (Cui et al., 1991; Norris et al., 1994). Furthermore, NB-UVB and MEL (coherent and incoherent) were both found to upregulate endothelin-1 (ET-1) release from keratinocytes, which is thought to play a role in UVB-related melanocyte synthesis and migration (Noborio, Kobayashi et al., 2006). This action is directly dependent on UVB radiation dose, and may account for the particular effectiveness of the 308 nm and

310-312 nm wavelengths (Noborio, Kobayashi et al., 2006). Also, the 308 nm wavelength of MEL is most specific for lymphocyte DNA alteration (de With and Greulich, 1995). The quantitative induction of T-cell apoptosis is greater with excimer laser (MEL) than with conventional BB- or NB-UVB phototherapies. It is thought that the capability to induce T-cell apoptosis is an indicator of clinical efficacy (Ozawa, Ferenczi et al., 1999). Furthermore, keratinocytes may be influenced to release other unidentified cytokines and factors, which suggests that UVB functions as an immunomodulator. This may support the theory of an autoimmune component in the pathogenesis of vitiligo.

4. BB-UVB phototherapy

Conventional BB-UVB phototherapy utilizes an artificial light source that emits in the radiation spectrum that extends from 280-320 nm (Cui, Shen et al., 1991; Norris, Horikawa et al., 1994). The pilot study of BB-UVB in vitiligo was reported in 1990, and observed that 57% of treated patients had excellent (>75%) repigmentation of vitiligo patches in a 52 week treatment period (Koster W, 1990). The investigators also noted its particular efficacy in facial lesions as well in skin types V and VI (Koster W, 1990). Little definitive evidence purports the use of BB-UVB in vitiligo, primarily due to the dominant and successful use of NB-UVB.

BB-UVB with vitamin supplementation was found to be effective in actively spreading vitiligo for inducing repigmentation when given 2-3 times weekly for 6-8 weeks (Don, Iuga et al., 2006). Although the role of vitamin supplementation was not substantiated in the outcome, this particular trial suggests that BB-UVB can be an effective treatment for vitiligo (Don, Iuga et al., 2006). Targeted BB-UVB and MEL were found to have nearly equal rates and degrees of repigmentation when evaluated after 8 treatments (Asawanonda, Kijluakiat et al., 2008).

Nearly 60% of patients had 80-100% repigmentation after 70 BB-UVB treatment sessions, a rate comparable to topical PUVA (55.6%) and NB-UVB (54.2%) treated patients in the same trial (El-Mofty, Mostafa et al., 2010). Other studies suggest that BB-UVB is less effective or had no effect compared to PUVA and NB-UVB phototherapy for the treatment of vitiligo (Hartmann, Lurz et al., 2005; Gawkrodger, Ormerod et al., 2008). Furthermore, targeted BB-UVB therapy was found to have limited effectiveness in vitiligo, and treatment-responsive areas were limited to the face (Akar, Tunca et al., 2009).

5. NB-UVB phototherapy

NB-UVB phototherapy utilizes the 311-313 nm radiation spectrum, which excludes the shorter and more erythmogenic wavelengths of BB- and natural (sunlight) UVB. It has been shown to be more effective than PUVA photochemotherapy, without the adverse side effect profile of psoralen (Table 1) (Bhatnagar, Kanwar et al., 2007; Yones, Palmer et al., 2007). Evidence-based guidelines suggest that NB-UVB should be used instead of PUVA in both adult and pediatric patients who have treatment-resistant disease, widespread involvement (BSA > 10-20%), or disease that severely affects quality of life (Ostovari, Passeron et al., 2004; Gawkrodger, Ormerod et al., 2008; Silverberg, 2010). Furthermore, NB-UVB is suggested as the best choice for generalized disease, with topical immunomodulators (*i.e.*, pimecrolimus cream or tacrolimus ointment) reserved for localized patches (Stinco, Piccirillo et al., 2009). Prognosis is significantly better in those with generalized vitiligo without acral involvement, and reportedly in females (El-Mofty, Mostafa et al., 2010). Less relevant predictors of clinical outcome include skin type, age, and previous response to phototherapy and other vitiligo treatments.

Author(s)	Country of Origin	Study Design	Number of Patients (Completing)	Frequency (per week)	Duration (weeks)	>75% Repigmentation	>50% Repigmentation	Notes
Yones, Palmer et al. 2007	England	Double-blind randomized	25				64%	Median number of treatments 97
Sitek, Loeb et al. 2007	Norway	Followup trial	31(11)		<52	35%		>75% repigmentation 2 years after treatment: 16%
Percivalle, Piccino et al. 2008	Italy	Longterm	53	2	<52	3.8%	32.05% (50-74%)	
Westerhof and Nieuweboer-Krobotova 1997	Netherlands	Open trial	51	2	12, 24, 36, 52	8 (12 weeks), 42 (24%), 49 (36%), 63 (52 weeks)		
Njoo, Bos et al. 2000	Netherlands	Open uncontrolled	51	2	<52	53		
Natta, Somsak et al. 2003	Thailand	Retrospective open analysis	60	2	20-104	33	42%	
Samson Yashar, Gielczyk et al. 2003	United States	Retrospective	77(71)	2-3		39		In 19-123 treatments, average 62
Hamzavi, Jain et al. 2004	Canada	Prospective randomized controlled	22	3	24			43% mean repigmentation, significant repigmentation by 8 weeks
Dogra and Kanwar 2004	India	Open uncontrolled	26(20)	3	<52	75		Mild-moderate: 20%
Kanwar, Dogra et al. 2005	India	Open uncontrolled	17(14)	3	<52	71.4		Mild-moderate: 14.3%
Chen, Hsu et al. 2005	Taiwan	Retrospective	72	2-3	<52	12.5	50-75%: 33.3%	7% with phototoxicity (burns)
Brazzelli, Prestinari et al. 2005	Italy	Open uncontrolled	10	2-3	<24	50		Average 48 treatments
Anbar, Westerhof et al. 2006	Netherlands	Open trial	97	2	32	48		76.3% face
Nicolai-dou, Antoniou et al. 2007	Greece	Open uncontrolled	70	2	<78	34.4% face, 7.4% body	50-75%: 13.1% face, 3% body	
Casacci, Thomas et al. 2007	France	Investigator blinded randomized halfside comparison	21	2	24	6%	31%	Less effective than MEL in head-to-head comparison

Table 1. NB-UVB Phototherapy Studies in Vitiligo

NB-UVB for vitiligo is most effective on the face and neck, followed by the trunk, and then upper extremities (Figure 3). Acral regions including the lower extremities, palms, and soles are more resistant to treatment. The reason has yet to be elucidated, but the regional density of hair follicles, which are reservoirs for melanocytes, are thought to play a role (Stinco, Piccirillo et al., 2009). In general, the repigmentation patterns in patients treated with NB-UVB are, in descending order, perifollicular (51.3%), then marginal, diffuse, and combined (Yang, Cho et al., 2010). However, the marginal pattern was observed to be the most common when >75% repigmentation occurred by 12 weeks of treatment (Yang, Cho et al., 2010).

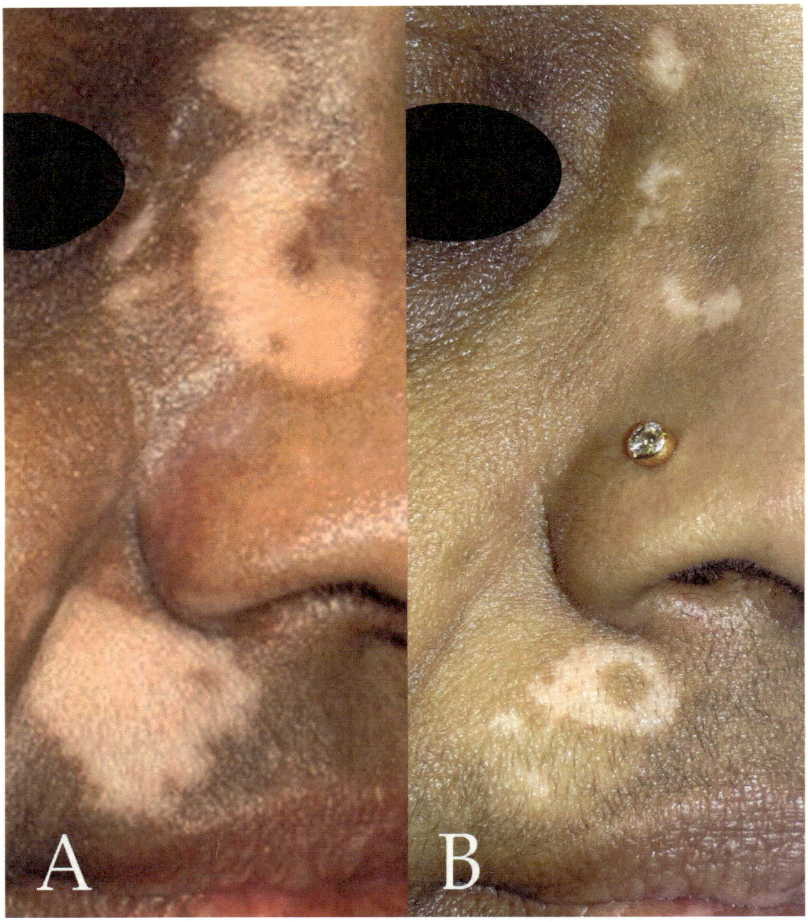

Fig. 3. A patient with facial vitiligo was treated with NB-UVB phototherapy three times weekly. A. The patient prior to initiating treatment. The patient was then started at 200 mJ based on standard protocol for Fitzpatrick skin type III. B. The patient with notable repigmentation after treatment 56 at a dose of 1001 mJ.

Patients should be counseled that, although these conventional phototherapies are quite effective for the head and neck region, they are less effective in the acral regions, which are commonly resistant areas, and in particular, the hands and feet. In addition, possible side effects, such as a predisposition to the development of skin malignancy, should be discussed. Phototherapy is ideal in patients who cannot tolerate or have failed other vitiligo treatments, elderly and pediatric patients, pregnant or lactating patients, and those with renal or hepatic dysfunction. It does not require systemic photosensitizers as in PUVA or other photochemotherapies. Administration is less cumbersome than PUVA, without the use of uncomfortable special protective eyewear that PUVA requires.

Home UVB therapy may be a valuable and convenient option for select patients. Patient-reported outcomes for home NB-UVB therapy and outpatient NB-UVB therapy revealed that they show similar clinical efficacy and safety profiles (Wind, Kroon et al., 2010). Home NB-UVB is convenient and can be cost-effective in certain situations. However, more reliable long-term follow-up data is needed to further justify home UVB therapy.

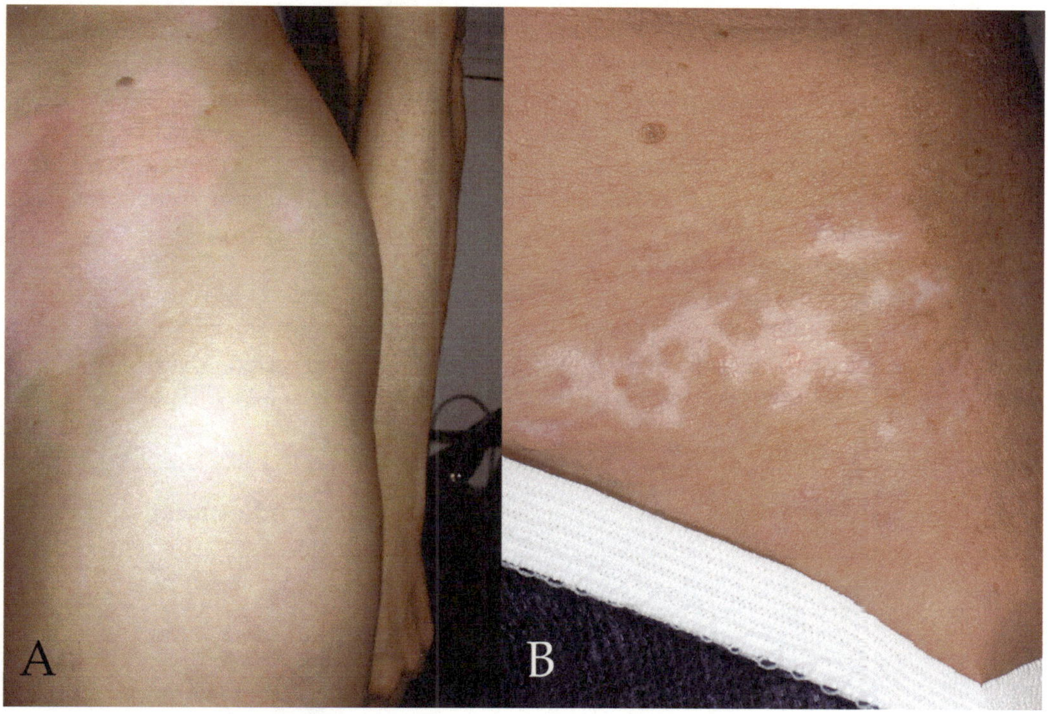

Fig. 4. A. Extensive vitiligo of the lower abdomen and hips. B. Repigmentation of vitiligo patches after 24 months of NB-UVB treatment.

6. Conventional UVB phototherapy administration and dosing

UVB phototherapy dosing is tailored to patient phototype (skin type). Other considerations include which and how much body surface area (BSA) is involved, the need for photoprotection of sensitive body areas such as the eyes or genitals, history of photosensitivity, use of photosensitizing drugs, previous UV irradiation history, and body surface area involvement, among other parameters. Both BB- and NB-UVB treatments are given in large whole-body chambers or cabins furnished with the designated high-intensity (BB-or NB-UVB) light tubes. NB-UVB should ideally occur three times a week with at least

24 hours (nonconsecutive days) in between treatments. The duration of treatment is often many months, and may be tapered down with time.

For both BB-UVB and NB-UVB, the starting, or induction, dose must be determined, which is generally the minimal erythema dose (MED). Then, between 50-70% of this MED, or erythmogenic dose, is used. After initial treatment, doses are increased by 5-20% of the previous dose if patient tolerates treatment without phototoxicity or pruritus. The MED may be difficult to determine in vitiligo due to small lesion sizes and the tedious testing process to determine MED. For NB-UVB treatment of vitiligo, patients can also be assumed to have Fitzgerald skin type I lesional skin, which has an MED of 400 millijoules per centimeters squared (mJ/cm^2) and further dosing is determined from this number.

The treatment cap for number of treatments that Fitzpatrick skin types I-III may receive is arbitrarily set at 200 treatments. While there is no set limit for skin types IV-VI, the recommendation for number of treatments should be based on clinician discretion and patient consent (Gawkrodger, Ormerod et al., 2008). However, treatment caps have yet to be defined but based on our experience, long-term NB-UVB is safe. In children, disease control and repigmentation is achieved with biweekly treatments for 12 weeks and continues for 12 months. At this point, 80% of pediatric patients have stabilization of disease (Silverberg, 2010). Serial photography is recommended every 2-3 months to monitor disease progress, failure to respond, and safety, according to well-developed protocols for adults (Gawkrodger, Ormerod et al., 2008).

For NB-UVB, the dosing protocol the authors recommend from decades of use in a dedicated academic phototherapy center, skin type is always assumed to be Type I, with initial dosing at 170 mJ, then increasing by 30 mJ at a time as tolerated. Missed treatments require dosage adjustment depending on number of days or weeks missed (Table 2).

Number of Missed Days	Dosage Adjustment
1-7	Increase per skin type I
8-11	Hold dose constant
12-20	Decrease by 25%
21-27	Decrease by 50%
28 or more	Start over

Table 2. NB-UVB Dosage Adjustments for Missed Treatment Days

Monitoring for side effects is crucial. The patient may report symptoms including burning, tightness, pruritus, and pain, among other phototoxicity-related complaints. The clinician may notice erythema or exacerbation of disease on physical examination. Focal erythema and tenderness can be managed by shielding affected areas until symptoms remit. The development of marked pain or blistering is an indication to reduce the previous dose of radiation by 25% and subsequently cautiously increasing dosage when there is no further adverse reaction.

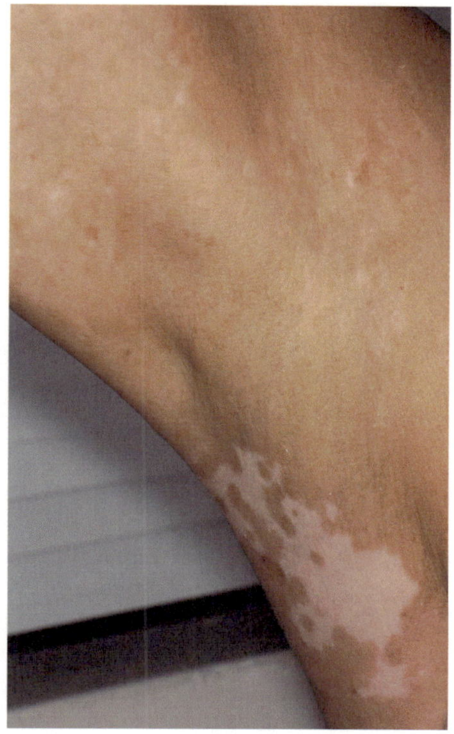

Fig. 5. Amelanotic patches of vitiligo in flexural areas undergoing involution NB-UVB therapy.

7. Monochromatic excimer light (MEL)

Xenon-chloride excimer (excited dimer) light is composed of the specific 308 nm wavelength, creating monochromatic radiation that is known as monochromatic excimer light, or MEL. The dimers are a halide (xenon) and noble gas (chloride) combination, which creates a high-energy unstable state, which is then translated into light radiation. It is clinically useful in the treatment of vitiligo, as well as other inflammatory skin diseases such as psoriasis, as well as mycosis fungoides. Sources of MEL include lamps, handheld devices, and in-office systems. These all emit MEL as *incoherent* light, similar to conventional UVB phototherapy in that it is nonselective for body treatment area and is non-targeted (as opposed to the excimer laser).

When a 308-nm MEL delivery system was used in vitiligo, half of lesions showed repigmentation at 2 weeks, and after an 8 week treatment period followed by a non-treatment 5 week observation period, all patients maintained their respective degrees of improvement (Table 3) (Chimento, Newland et al., 2008). In general, patients who respond to MEL do so at the beginning, otherwise they do not respond at all (Leone, Iacovelli et al., 2003). MEL has also successfully treated previously NB-UVB refractory disease, and has been shown to be more effective and quicker than conventional NB-UVB (Leone, Iacovelli et al., 2003; Le Duff, Fontas et al., 2010). In a head-to-head study in which patients served as their own controls, the 308-nm excimer laser and MEL lamp had similar efficacy, although the lamp induces more erythema (Le Duff, Fontas et al., 2010). In addition, the use of lower power density reduces the risk of adverse events.

Author(s)	Country of Origin	Study Design	Number of Patients (Completing)	Number of Patches	Frequency (per week)	Duration (weeks)	>75% Repigmentation	>50% Repigmentation	Notes
Saraceno, Nistico et al. 2009	Italy	Open prospective	48(45)		1	12	62.5% (+ PO vitamin E) 56.25% (+ khellin 4% ointment)	12.5 (50-75%) 31.25%	Control group 18.75% (50-75) (+ PO vitamin E)
Chimento, Newland et al. 2008	United States		10			10			Repigmentation in in 50% of patients at 2 weeks, maintained in follow-up period of 5 weeks
Xiang 2008	China		36 (active) 41 (stable)	91, 110			29.7 (active), 30.9% (stable)		2.6% relapse rate in 2 year follow-up
Lu-Yan, Wen-wen et al. 2006	China	Double blinded within patient controlled	38(35)	70	1	12	Excellent: 5.7% (+placebo), (+TAC 25.7%)		
Casacci, Thomas et al. 2007	France	Investigator blinded randomized half-side comparison	21		2	24	37.5%	25%	Superior to NB-UVB in head-to-head comparison
Le Duff, Fontas et al. 2010	France	Randomized monocentric	20(17)	104	2	12	38%	15%	Equal to excimer laser in head-to-head comparison

Table 3. MEL Phototherapy Studies in Vitiligo

The advantage of MEL includes the ability to irradiate larger body surface areas rather than the confined target areas of lasers and that it can be used to treat the entire body at once. It can also be customized to treat certain patches, has the perks of shorter treatment times, frequency, and total treatment duration, which in turn can lead to increased patient compliance (Leone, Iacovelli et al., 2003).

8. Excimer laser

The use of laser (*l*ight *a*mplification by *s*timulated *e*mission of *r*adiation) technology in dermatology was introduced in the mid-1980s and has since been applied to vitiligo therapy. The specific 308 nm wavelength utilized by MEL also comes in a *coherent,* or targeted format, which is administered by laser.

The excimer laser is a well-tolerated, effective treatment that induces quicker repigmentation than other forms of vitiligo therapy (Spencer, Nossa et al., 2002). It is thought to share a similar mechanism of action as other UVB therapies, as evidenced by treated vitiligo patches that undergo the same repigmentation patterns observed in conventional NB-UVB phototherapy (Yang, Cho et al., 2010).

Vitiligo patch location and duration of disease are thought to be factors in the efficacy and response to excimer laser (Hofer, Hassan et al., 2005; Zhang, He et al., 2010) The face, neck, and to a lesser extent, the trunk, are more sensitive, or responsive, to laser treatment than more resistant areas which have been identified as the acral areas of the extremities and bony prominences (Ostovari, Passeron et al., 2004). Clinical outcome is dependent on the total number of laser treatments, not treatment frequency. However, repigmentation is induced quickest with increased frequency: optimal treatment occurs three times weekly, followed by twice weekly treatments (Hofer, Hassan et al., 2005; Shen, Gao et al., 2007). Once weekly treatment is also acceptable and effective, and may increase patient compliance due to decreased clinic visit frequency (Xiang, 2008). The 308-nm excimer laser is also effective and safe treatment for pediatric patients, in particular those with localized disease (Cho, Zheng et al., 2011).

Compared with conventional NB-UVB phototherapy, the excimer laser is not only more efficacious, allowing for lower cumulative dosing and faster clearance, but also spares normal unaffected skin from carcinogenic UV radiation exposure. The laser light intensity is much greater than conventional NB-UVB phototherapy and its energy is emitted in nanoseconds (rather than minutes). It is suggested that the increased efficacy in inducing T-cell apoptosis allows for greater clinical efficacy of the laser than other conventional light therapies.

Side effects are generally well-tolerated, and are usually due to phototoxicity, *i.e.*, erythema, hyperpigmentation, erosions, and blisters (Housman, Pearce et al., 2004). Patients with Fitzpatrick skin type 1 may be prone to frequent blistering, especially with the usage of supra-erythmogenic laser therapy. Subsequent conservative dosing, may not achieve any more benefit than general UVB phototherapy regimens (Gattu, Pang et al., 2010). In addition, it can be used for patients with phobia of the light box or phototherapy unit, and may be more tolerable for children (Lapidoth, Adatto et al., 2007) However, the excimer laser is currently limited to outpatient use, which requires frequent clinic visits over a short time duration, which can lead to low patient compliance (Kemeny, Csoma et al., 2010).

Authors	Country of Origin	Number of Patients (Completing Study)	Number of Patches	Frequency (per week)	Duration (weeks)	Repigmentation Results	Notes
Zhang, He et al. 2010	China	36	44	2	15	>75%: 61.4%	30 treatments
Sassi, Cazzaniga et al. 2008	Italy	84(76)		2	12	100%: 4.7% (+steroid 21.4%) >75%: 16.6% (+steroid 21.4%)	Monotherapy compared with combination topical steroid
Baltas, Csoma et al. 2002	Hungary	6(4)	4	2	24	>75%: 75%	No depigmentation at 3 month follow-up
Hadi, Spencer et al. 2004	United States	32	55	2	15	>75%: 51%	Results seen at 30 treatments; no depigmentation at 1 month follow-up
Leone, Iacovelli et al. 2003	Italy	37(36)		2	<24	>75%: 12% at 12 weeks, 18% at 24 weeks 50+%: 21% at 12 weeks, 16% at 24 weeks	
Al-Otaibi, Zadeh et al. 2009	Kuwait	34(29)		2		>75%: 20.7% 43.75% face 33.4% trunk 50+%: 41.4%	25 treatments
Cho, Zheng et al. 2011	South Korea	30(30)	40	2	13	>75%: 12.5%	
Spencer, Nossa et al. 2002	United States	12	6	3	4	82%: 11 patches in 12 treatments 57%: 23 patches in +6 treatments	Time to repigmentation 2-4 weeks
Taneja, Trehan et al. 2003	United States	18	15	2	30	>75%: 33%	100% face
Choi, Park et al. 2004	South Korea		50	2	15	>75%: 15.7%	33% face and neck
Ostovari, Passeron et al. 2004	France	35	31	2	12	>75%: 27%	57% face, neck, trunk
Esposito, Soda et al. 2004	Italy	24	24	2	36	>75%: 29%	

Authors	Country of Origin	Number of Patients (Completing Study)	Number of Patches	Frequency (per week)	Duration (weeks)	Repigmentation Results	Notes
Hong, Park et al. 2005	South Korea	8	8	2	10	>75%: 0%	
Hofer, Hassan et al. 2006	Austria	25	24	3	6-10	>75%: 25% (face, trunk, arm, leg)	
Hadi, Tinio et al. 2006	United States	97	221			100%: 25.5% >75%: 50.6% >50%: 64.3%	
Passeron, Ostovari et al. 2004	France	14	20 monotherapy , 23 + Tacrolimus	2	12	>75%: 20%	>75%: 70% (+ Tacrolimus)
Kawalek, Spencer et al. 2004	United States	8	6	3	8-10	>75%: 20%	>75%: 50% (+ Tacrolimus)
Le Duff, Fontas et al. 2010	France	20(17)	104	2	12	>75%: 42%, >50%: 15%	Equal to MEL in head-to-head comparison

Table 4. Excimer Laser Phototherapy Studies in Vitiligo

9. Microphototherapy

Focused microphototherapy was developed in 1999, and utilizes UVB light in the 280-315 nm spectrum. This form of UVB therapy uses a dark-colored pad with perforations to focus light only on vitiligo patches using an optical fiber and hood. Its efficacy in vitiligo has shown promising results (Lotti, Menchini et al., 1999; Lotti, Tripo et al., 2009). Treatment protocol begins with daily treatment for a week, then tapered down to a few times a week, and finally, twice monthly. Half of patients show a moderate response to treatment, and a quarter of patients have excellent (>75%) repigmentation. However, focused microphototherapy is laborious, requiring expensive tools and training to perform the procedures.

10. Combination therapy

The UVB phototherapy modalities can be combined with other vitiligo treatments. These include combinations with topical preparations including immunomodulators such as pimecrolimus and tacrolimus, immunosuppresants such as corticosteroids, and vitamin D analogues. Systemic medications can also be part of combination therapy, and these include supplements such as antioxidants as well as systemic corticosteroids.

10.1 Pimecrolimus

Pimecrolimus is a calcineurin inhibitor and immunomodulator available as a cream. It is generally well-tolerated and safe for long-term use. This topical formulation is used once to twice daily on vitiligo patches. Pimecrolimus inhibits T cell activation; however, data on melanocyte function are lacking (Dawid, Veensalu et al., 2006). Although already useful as monotherapy, it is also able to enhance phototherapy efficacy. NB-UVB works better if combined with pimecrolimus 1% cream (64.3%) rather than photomonotherapy (25.1%) on facial lesions (Elgoweini and Nour El Din, 2009). Pediatric patients also tolerate this combination well, with excellent repigmentation on the face, and with varying degrees of effectiveness on all body parts (Elgoweini and Nour El Din, 2009). Side effects are tolerated well and generally limited to phototoxic effects such as mild discomfort, neurosis, and erythema. Furthermore, pimecrolimus may sometimes exacerbate symptoms after phototherapy, which include blistering and pruritus (Hui-Lan, Xiao-Yan et al., 2009).

10.2 Tacrolimus

Tacrolimus, like pimecrolimus, is a calcineurin inhibitor and immunomodulator in an ointment formulation that is used once to twice daily for vitiligo and is an option for long-term management. It is empirically used in vitiligo due to its ability to increase melanocyte proliferation as well as stem cell factors, and down-regulate a number of interleukins, interferon-gamma, tumor necrosis factor-alpha, and granulocyte monocyte-colony stimulating factor (Grimes, Soriano et al., 2002; Lan, Chen et al., 2005). Tacrolimus ointment (0.1%) and NB-UVB combination treatment is more effective than NB-UVB monotherapy and the effect of tacrolimus is dose-dependent (Nordal, Guleng et al., 2011). The efficacy of tacrolimus and excimer laser is also additive; repigmentation is achieved quicker with total lower cumulative laser dosage (Passeron, Ostovari et al., 2004). Side effects due to tacrolimus-phototherapy dual therapy include itching, formication, erythema, and soreness.

Either pimecrolimus or tacrolimus with UVB as combination therapy are best used in sun-exposed areas due to better treatment outcomes with combination therapy than non-exposed skin (Stinco, Piccirillo et al., 2009). There is a non-significant difference in efficacy between pimecrolimus and tacrolimus, although pimecrolimus may be slightly more effective due to its lipophilic properties that enable it to penetrate depigmented epidermis better than tacrolimus (Stinco, Piccirillo et al., 2009).

10.3 Vitamin D analogues

Calcipotriol, or calcipotriene, and tacalcitol are synthetic vitamin D3 (calcitriol) analogues which bind to vitamin D receptors in the epidermis and affect melanocyte and keratinocyte maturation. These receptors are also on T cells. Studies found that combination calcipotriol and NB-UVB therapy was not superior to NB-UVB alone (Ada, Sahin et al., 2005; Hartmann, Lurz et al., 2005). Similar findings were found when calcipotriene ointment and NB-UVB three times weekly were combined (Kullavanijaya and Lim, 2004). The combination of the 308 nm excimer laser and calcipotriol also did not seem to be superior to excimer laser alone in a small trial in patients who served as their own controls (Goldinger, Dummer et al., 2007). However, tacalcitol and 308 nm excimer laser treatment is superior to the laser alone; and allows for quicker improvement into vitiligo patches with lower cumulative dosing (Lu-yan, Wen-wen et al., 2006).

10.4 Corticosteroids

Topical corticosteroids have some value in vitiligo treatment but with the high risk of side effects, most commonly skin atrophy, as well as striae, erythema, and absorption near the eyes which poses a risk for glaucoma candidates (Gawkrodger, Ormerod et al., 2008). They should be reserved for short-term (< 2 months) use only. Recalcitrant vitiligo of the face and neck may benefit from the combination of excimer laser phototherapy with topical hydrocortisone 17-butyrate cream.This was observed to have induce >75% repigmentation of vitiligo involvement in 3 months (Sassi, Cazzaniga et al., 2008). Systemic immunosuppression to prevent progression of vitiligo using oral corticosteroids is not recommended for treatment due to the high risk of side effects, although used by some clinicians for active or rapidly progressing vitiligo. Furthermore, the additive effect of oral steroids to either NB- or BB-UVB phototherapy is minimal (Rath, Kar et al., 2008).

10.5 Vitamins & antioxidants

Supplemental vitamins and minerals are popular remedies and adjuncts for vitiligo therapy. It is thought that there is a relationship between vitiligo pathogenesis and oxidative stress (Gawkrodger, Ormerod et al., 2008). In conjunction with vitamin C (500mg twice daily), vitamin B12 (1,000 micrograms twice daily), and folic acid (5 mg twice daily), BB-UVB had a significant clinically efficacious outcome in actively spreading vitiligo. Vitamin supplementation was used hypothetically and the investigators could only imply that BB-UVB could be effective for vitiligo and the role of vitamins was unclear (Don, Iuga et al., 2006).

In combination with NB-UVB, oral vitamin E supplementation (400 IU) was shown to augment therapy by hypothetically preventing lipid peroxidation of melanocytes and reducing phototherapy-related erythema (Elgoweini and Nour El Din, 2009). The use of vitamin A supplements has also been studied, but its use with NB-UVB is not supported (Elgoweini and Nour El Din, 2009).

10.6 L-phenylalanine

Phenylalanine (L-phenylalanine) supplementation is thought to supply precursors for melanin production. It is an essential amino acid that is the precursor to tyrosine in melanin synthesis by hydroxylation and thereby turns into melanin. Although naturally occurring in the diet, supplementation and UV radiation administration is said to have some clinical value in vitiligo without any reports of serious adverse effects (Schulpis, Antoniou et al., 1989).

10.7 Pseudocatalase

Pseudocatalase is a low molecular-weight manganese complex that serves as a substitute for naturally occurring catalase, which is thought to be inactivated in vitiligo by hydrogen peroxide accumulation in the epidermis. It is used in combination with UVB and climatotherapy, the latter which is the physical relocation of the patient to an area with a climate ideal or more suitable to a disease, in this case, vitiligo. Topically applied pseudocatalase and calcium used twice daily with twice weekly UVB phototherapy had a 90% repigmentation rate in an uncontrolled clinical trial. Initial results were seen in 8-16 weeks. In comparison to NB-UVB monotherapy, pseudocatalase and NB-UVB combination treatment showed clinically significant results, and was superior, with >75% of treatment sites with repigmentation vs. 70% in NB-UVB monotherapy (Schallreuter and Rokos, 2007). Side effects include pruritus, hyperhidrosis, and hyperpigmentation.

10.8 Tetrahydrocurcuminoid

Tetrahydrocurcuminoid (THC) is a derivative of curcumin (diferuloymethane) which is a compound collected from the roots of tumeric (*Curcuma longa).* Based on the theory of combatting oxidative stress as a treatment for vitiligo, curcumin was the anti-inflammatory agent investigated. Curcumoid cream (with the main active ingredient being THC) applied twice daily along with targeted NB-UVB twice weekly had higher repigmentation scores than phototherapy alone, although this was not statistically significant (Asawanonda and Klahan, 2010).

10.9 Khellin

Khellin is a furanochromone (dimethoxy-4, 9 methyl-7 oxo-5 5-H-Furo [3,2-G]-4H chromone) that is chemically similar to psoralen, which is the basis of PUVA photochemotherapy. It is clinically safer and less damaging to cellular DNA than psoralen. Khellin stimulates melanocyte activation, proliferation, migration, and melanogenesis (Carlie, Ntusi et al., 2003). Compared with MEL monotherapy, combination MEL and topical khellin 4% ointment had more > 75% repigmentation rates than MEL alone (25% vs. 56.25%) (Saraceno, Nistico et al., 2009). Response is best in acute patches of the face, neck, and knees (Saraceno, Nistico et al., 2009).

10.10 Microphototherapy

The use of 311-nm narrow-band microphototherapy has been augmented with tacrolimus 0.1% ointment twice a day, pimecrolimus 1% cream twice a day, betamethasone dipropionate 0.05% cream twice a day, calcipotriol ointment 50 micrograms/gram twice a day, and 10% l-phenylalanine cream twice a day. Of these combinations, the 311-nm narrow-band UVB microfocused phototherapy with 0.05% betamethasone dipropionate cream gives the best repigmentation rate. In the latter treatment, the only short-term side effect is skin atrophy due to the corticosteroid cream (Lotti, Buggiani et al., 2008).

10.11 Surgery

Surgery may be an option for vitiligo treatment for disease refractory to conventional medical treatment. The use of split-skin grafting consists of harvesting the epidermis and part of the dermis from a normally concealed donor site (such as the inner thigh) for use on a mechanically manipulated (*e.g.*, via dermabrasion) recipient area. Use of the 308 nm excimer laser for 32 treatments that were initiated 2 weeks post-surgery had a 100% response rate in patients by the end of therapy. Follow-up after one year showed even greater improvement in recipient sites (Al-Mutairi, Manchanda et al., 2010).

Punch grafting followed by use of NB-UVB also results in better cosmetic outcome of surgical sites, with repigmentation in the majority of cases (Lahiri, Malakar et al., 2006). It is thought that adjunctive NB-UVB is an efficient, safe, and cost-effective addition to surgical procedures for vitiligo.

11. Adverse effects and long-term usage

Short-term adverse effects related to UVB phototherapy are mostly related to phototoxicity which includes burning, pruritus, xerosis, pain, blistering, as well as increased susceptibility to cutaneous herpes simplex virus infections. These can be managed with early identification and topical corticosteroids as well as the judicious use of systemic steroids and anti-inflammatory agents in serious cases. Overaggressive treatment resulting in phototoxic reactions (*i.e.*, erythema) can lead to koebnerization.

Long-term UVB exposure is associated with photodamage and photoaging, and is a carcinogen with the potential to increase long-term risk of malignancy (Gonzaga, 2009). At baseline, vitiligo patients with Fitzpatrick skin types I and II have a non-statistically significant increased risk of nonmelanoma skin cancer than the general population; however, this is not reported in more pigmented skin types (type III and above) (Hexsel, Eide et al., 2009).

In Caucasian-based population studies, PUVA is an established risk factor for NMSC, particularly with long-term therapy in patients with skin types I-II patients (Stern and Laird, 1994). This risk has been appreciated as early as within a 2-year follow-up period (Stern and Laird, 1994). It is the strongest predictor of squamous cell carcinoma (SCC) risk, the latter of which is also influenced by male gender, having skin types I-II, residence in southern regions, as well as the use of high-dose methotrexate and/or cyclosporin (Lim and Stern, 2005). PUVA only modestly increases BCC risk, which is also increased by male gender and exposure to high dose tar and/or methotrexate. NMSC due to PUVA use is modestly increased with high UVB exposure (>300 treatments) limited to less than 100 PUVA treatments, however these appear on usually non-sun exposed anatomic sites (Lim and Stern, 2005). However, the carcinogenic risk of PUVA in non-Caucasians, in particular, Asian and Arabian-African populations, is not substantiated (Murase, Lee et al., 2005). The analysis of the effect of ethnicity on PUVA risk of 4,294 long-term non-Caucasian PUVA patients with at least a 5-year follow-up implied that pigmented skin and ethnic skin types may confer photoprotection (Murase, Lee et al., 2005). Therefore, although the carcinogenic risks of PUVA therapy must be seriously considered in Caucasian vitiligo patients, vitiligo patients with skin of color may consider PUVA therapy with more assurance.

Author	Country	Phototherapy Type	Number of Patients	Person Years	Duration of Follow-up	Number of Treatments (average)	Skin Type	Results
Jo, Kwon et al. 2010	Korea	NB-UVB	445	1274	34.4 months	33.6	III-V	No increased skin cancer risk
Black and Gavin 2006	England	NB-UVB	484			18	I-II (92%)	As expected per general population
Hearn, Kerr et al. 2008	Scotland	NB-UVB	4665	24,753	6 months – 22 years	29 (median)	I (23%), II (47%) III (27%)	NB-UVB monotherapy no increase in NMSC or melanoma; NB-UVB + PUVA no increase in SCC or melanoma, BCC incre-ased (27 vs. 14.1 in general population)
Man, Crombie et al. 2005	Scotland	NB-UVB	1908		4 years (median), <13 years	23 (median)	I-III (BCC patie-nts)	No increase risk SCC or melanoma; excess BCC noted, but 60+% were diagnosed at referral
Weischer, Blum et al. 2004	Germany	BB-UVB	69/195	BB-UVB 533	BB-UVB 68.3	BB-UVB 17.8	Only 2 patie-nts with V noted	BB-UVB no increase NMSC or MM
		NB-UVB	126/195	NB-UVB 726	NB-UVB 93.6	NB-UVB 44		NB-UVB no increase NMSC, 1 case MM in first year of treatment
Lim and Stern 2005	United States	UVB	1154/ 1380	27,928	>14 years	403	I-II, III-V as refe-rence group	UVB >300 vs <300: increase SCC IRR 1.37, increase BCC 1.45
		PUVA	1380	27,928	>14 years		I-II, III-V as refe-rence group	PUVA <100 + UVB (>300): increase SCC IRR 2.75, increase BCC 3
Pittelkow, Perry et al. 1981	United States	UVB	280		25 years			No increased risk NMSC
Larko and Swanbeck 1982	Sweden	UVB	85					Prevalence premalignant and malignancy cutaneous malignancies: 5.9% in treated vs. 10.1% in controls

Table 5. Phototherapy Follow-up in Dermatology Patients and Carcinogenic Risk

When comparing UVB and PUVA carcinogenic risk, a single PUVA increases risk 7 times more than a single UVB treatment (Lim and Stern, 2005). Even with a history of PUVA therapy, patients who had less than 300 treatments of UVB had no appreciable increase in NMSC risk (Lim and Stern, 2005). Available data on NB-UVB therapy has not consistently identified a significant increase in NMSC when compared to the general population (Table 4). The majority of follow-up data was primarily taken from Caucasian populations, but the same conclusion has been drawn in non-Caucasians with skin types III-V (Jo, Kwon et al., 2010). An increased risk of BCC was noted in two Scottish studies, one with NB-UVB monotherapy, and the other with a history of both NB-UVB and PUVA usage (Stern and Laird, 1994; Man, Crombie et al., 2005). However, the temporal relationship between tumor diagnosis and phototherapy makes a relationship between therapy and cancer unlikely in either study (Stern and Laird, 1994; Man, Crombie et al., 2005). In addition, it is common to use topical pimecrolimus and/or tacrolimus as adjuncts to NB-UVB. Topical pimecrolimus and tacrolimus have not been found to increase risk of NMSC in adults. Therefore, even in combination with NB-UVB, there should be no cumulative carcinogenic effect. Therefore, UVB, in particular NB-UVB, may be the phototherapy option with the least carcinogenic risk in all skin types.

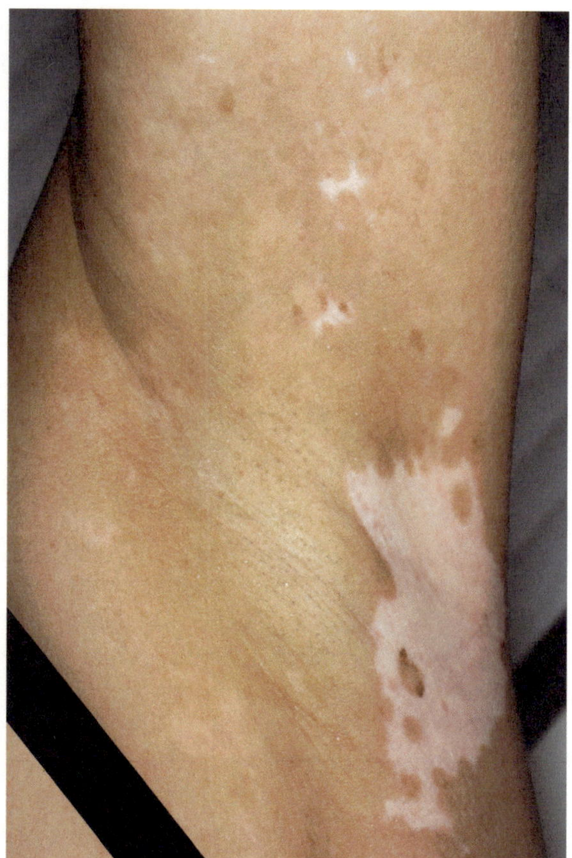

Fig. 6. NB-UVB is an effective treatment modality for vitiligo. Short term adverse effects are primarily related to phototoxicity. Long-term carcinogenic risk may not differ greatly from the general population.

Due to lack of long-term phototherapy research data specifically in vitiligo, it is difficult to wholly substantiate any claims regarding potential risk. Available phototherapy follow-up data was drawn from patients treated with a variety of photoresponsive dermatoses, which includes vitiligo, despite lack of quantification of vitiligo cases. Further research specifically on carcinogenic risk in vitiligo is needed.

12. Conclusion

Although multiple management options exist for vitiligo, UVB phototherapy is generally the treatment of choice as it is not only effective but has a favorable risk-to-benefit ratio. Conventional BB- and NB-UVB is widely available and useful particularly in widespread disease, although NB-UVB has been more extensively studied with proven efficacy. The development of MEL has provided options for both generalized and limited disease and is available in a variety of treatment systems. MEL has also been applied to laser therapy, which is growing in popularity due to the benefits of quicker treatment duration, increased efficacy, and a better risk-to-benefit ratio compared to conventional phototherapy techniques. Combination therapies are also useful and may provide quicker regimentation and treat vitiligo with an additive mechanism of action than UVB phototherapy. Advances in technology may lead to the continuing use of UVB phototherapy as a treatment for vitiligo through the development of sophisticated devices and delivery systems as well as innovative application methods. These will provide increased therapeutic options for all vitiligo patients, particularly those with refractory disease.

13. References

Ada, S., S. Sahin, et al. (2005). No additional effect of topical calcipotriol on narrow-band UVB phototherapy in patients with generalized vitiligo. *Photodermatol Photoimmunol Photomed* 21(2): 79-83.

Akar, A., M. Tunca, et al. (2009). Broadband targeted UVB phototherapy for localized vitiligo: a retrospective study. *Photodermatol Photoimmunol Photomed* 25(3): 161-163.

Al-Mutairi, N., Y. Manchanda, et al. (2010). Long-term results of split-skin grafting in combination with excimer laser for stable vitiligo. *Dermatol Surg* 36(4): 499-505.

Al-Otaibi, S. R., V. B. Zadeh, et al. (2009). Using a 308-nm excimer laser to treat vitiligo in Asians. *Acta Dermatovenerol Alp Panonica Adriat* 18(1): 13-19.

Anbar, T. S., W. Westerhof, et al. (2006). Evaluation of the effects of NB-UVB in both segmental and non-segmental vitiligo affecting different body sites. *Photodermatol Photoimmunol Photomed* 22(3): 157-163.

Asawanonda, P., J. Kijluakiat, et al. (2008). Targeted broadband ultraviolet b phototherapy produces similar responses to targeted narrowband ultraviolet B phototherapy for vitiligo: a randomized, double-blind study. *Acta Derm Venereol* 88(4): 376-381.

Asawanonda, P. and S. O. Klahan (2010). Tetrahydrocurcuminoid cream plus targeted narrowband UVB phototherapy for vitiligo: a preliminary randomized controlled study. *Photomed Laser Surg* 28(5): 679-684.

Baltas, E., Z. Csoma, et al. (2002). Treatment of vitiligo with the 308-nm xenon chloride excimer laser. *Arch Dermatol* 138(12): 1619-1620.

Bhatnagar, A., A. J. Kanwar, et al. (2007). Comparison of systemic PUVA and NB-UVB in the treatment of vitiligo: an open prospective study. *J Eur Acad Dermatol Venereol* 21(5): 638-642.

Black, R. J. and A. T. Gavin (2006). Photocarcinogenic risk of narrowband ultraviolet B (TL-01) phototherapy: early follow-up data. *Br J Dermatol* 154(3): 566-567.

Bonis, B., L. Kemeny, et al. (1997). 308 nm UVB excimer laser for psoriasis. *Lancet* 350(9090): 1522.

Brazzelli, V., F. Prestinari, et al. (2005). Useful treatment of vitiligo in 10 children with UV-B narrowband (311 nm). *Pediatr Dermatol* 22(3): 257-261.

Carlie, G., N. B. Ntusi, et al. (2003). KUVA (khellin plus ultraviolet A) stimulates proliferation and melanogenesis in normal human melanocytes and melanoma cells in vitro. *Br J Dermatol* 149(4): 707-717.

Casacci, M., P. Thomas, et al. (2007). Comparison between 308-nm monochromatic excimer light and narrowband UVB phototherapy (311-313 nm) in the treatment of vitiligo--a multicentre controlled study. *J Eur Acad Dermatol Venereol* 21(7): 956-963.

Chen, G. Y., M. M. Hsu, et al. (2005). Narrow-band UVB treatment of vitiligo in Chinese. *J Dermatol* 32(10): 793-800.

Chimento, S. M., M. Newland, et al. (2008). A pilot study to determine the safety and efficacy of monochromatic excimer light in the treatment of vitiligo. *J Drugs Dermatol* 7(3): 258-263.

Cho, S., Z. Zheng, et al. (2011). The 308-nm excimer laser: a promising device for the treatment of childhood vitiligo. *Photodermatol Photoimmunol Photomed* 27(1): 24-29.

Choi, K. H., J. H. Park, et al. (2004). Treatment of Vitiligo with 308-nm xenon-chloride excimer laser: therapeutic efficacy of different initial doses according to treatment areas. *J Dermatol* 31(4): 284-292.

Cui, J., L. Y. Shen, et al. (1991). Role of hair follicles in the repigmentation of vitiligo. *J Invest Dermatol* 97(3): 410-416.

Dawid, M., M. Veensalu, et al. (2006). Efficacy and safety of pimecrolimus cream 1% in adult patients with vitiligo: results of a randomized, double-blind, vehicle-controlled study. *J Dtsch Dermatol Ges* 4(11): 942-946.

de With, A. and K. O. Greulich (1995). Wavelength dependence of laser-induced DNA damage in lymphocytes observed by single-cell gel electrophoresis. *J Photochem Photobiol B* 30(1): 71-76.

Dogra, S. and A. J. Kanwar (2004). Narrow band UVB phototherapy in dermatology. *Indian J Dermatol Venereol Leprol* 70(4): 205-209.

Don, P., A. Iuga, et al. (2006). Treatment of vitiligo with broadband ultraviolet B and vitamins. *Int J Dermatol* 45(1): 63-65.

El-Mofty, M., W. Z. Mostafa, et al. (2010). A large scale analytical study on efficacy of different photo(chemo)therapeutic modalities in the treatment of psoriasis, vitiligo and mycosis fungoides. *Dermatol Ther* 23(4): 428-434.

Elgoweini, M. and N. Nour El Din (2009). Response of vitiligo to narrowband ultraviolet B and oral antioxidants. *J Clin Pharmacol* 49(7): 852-855.

Esposito, M., R. Soda, et al. (2004). Treatment of vitiligo with the 308 nm excimer laser. *Clin Exp Dermatol* 29(2): 133-137.

Gattu, S., M. L. Pang, et al. (2010). Pilot evaluation of supra-erythemogenic phototherapy with excimer laser in the treatment of patients with moderate to severe plaque psoriasis. *J Dermatolog Treat* 21(1): 54-60.

Gawkrodger, D. J., A. D. Ormerod, et al. (2008). Guideline for the diagnosis and management of vitiligo. *Br J Dermatol* 159(5): 1051-1076.

Goldinger, S. M., R. Dummer, et al. (2007). Combination of 308-nm xenon chloride excimer laser and topical calcipotriol in vitiligo. *J Eur Acad Dermatol Venereol* 21(4): 504-508.

Gonzaga, E. R. (2009). Role of UV light in photodamage, skin aging, and skin cancer: importance of photoprotection. *Am J Clin Dermatol* 10 Suppl 1: 19-24.

Grimes, P. E., T. Soriano, et al. (2002). Topical tacrolimus for repigmentation of vitiligo. *J Am Acad Dermatol* 47(5): 789-791.

Hadi, S., P. Tinio, et al. (2006). Treatment of vitiligo using the 308-nm excimer laser. *Photomed Laser Surg* 24(3): 354-357.

Hadi, S. M., J. M. Spencer, et al. (2004). The use of the 308-nm excimer laser for the treatment of vitiligo. *Dermatol Surg* 30(7): 983-986.

Hamzavi, I., H. Jain, et al. (2004). Parametric modeling of narrowband UV-B phototherapy for vitiligo using a novel quantitative tool: the Vitiligo Area Scoring Index. *Arch Dermatol* 140(6): 677-683.

Hartmann, A., C. Lurz, et al. (2005). Narrow-band UVB311 nm vs. broad-band UVB therapy in combination with topical calcipotriol vs. placebo in vitiligo. *Int J Dermatol* 44(9): 736-742.

Hearn, R. M., A. C. Kerr, et al. (2008). Incidence of skin cancers in 3867 patients treated with narrow-band ultraviolet B phototherapy. *Br J Dermatol* 159(4): 931-935.

Hexsel, C. L., M. J. Eide, et al. (2009). Incidence of nonmelanoma skin cancer in a cohort of patients with vitiligo. *J Am Acad Dermatol* 60(6): 929-933.

Hofer, A., A. S. Hassan, et al. (2005). Optimal weekly frequency of 308-nm excimer laser treatment in vitiligo patients. *Br J Dermatol* 152(5): 981-985.

Hofer, A., A. S. Hassan, et al. (2006). The efficacy of excimer laser (308 nm) for vitiligo at different body sites. *J Eur Acad Dermatol Venereol* 20(5): 558-564.

Hong, S. B., H. H. Park, et al. (2005). Short-term effects of 308-nm xenon-chloride excimer laser and narrow-band ultraviolet B in the treatment of vitiligo: a comparative study. *J Korean Med Sci* 20(2): 273-278.

Housman, T. S., D. J. Pearce, et al. (2004). A maintenance protocol for psoriasis plaques cleared by the 308 nm excimer laser. *J Dermatolog Treat* 15(2): 94-97.

Hui-Lan, Y., H. Xiao-Yan, et al. (2009). Combination of 308-nm excimer laser with topical pimecrolimus for the treatment of childhood vitiligo. *Pediatr Dermatol* 26(3): 354-356.

Jo, S. J., H. H. Kwon, et al. (2010). No Evidence for Increased Skin Cancer Risk in Koreans with Skin Phototypes III-V Treated with Narrowband UVB Phototherapy. *Acta Derm Venereol.*

Kanwar, A. J., S. Dogra, et al. (2005). Narrow-band UVB for the treatment of vitiligo: an emerging effective and well-tolerated therapy. *Int J Dermatol* 44(1): 57-60.

Kawalek, A. Z., J. M. Spencer, et al. (2004). Combined excimer laser and topical tacrolimus for the treatment of vitiligo: a pilot study. *Dermatol Surg* 30(2 Pt 1): 130-135.

Kemeny, L., Z. Csoma, et al. (2010). Targeted phototherapy of plaque-type psoriasis using ultraviolet B-light-emitting diodes. *Br J Dermatol* 163(1): 167-173.

Koster W, W. A. (1990). Phototherapy with UVB in vitiligo. *J Hautkr* 65: 1022-1024.

Kullavanijaya, P. and H. W. Lim (2004). Topical calcipotriene and narrowband ultraviolet B in the treatment of vitiligo. *Photodermatol Photoimmunol Photomed* 20(5): 248-251.

Lahiri, K., S. Malakar, et al. (2006). Repigmentation of vitiligo with punch grafting and narrow-band UV-B (311 nm)--a prospective study. *Int J Dermatol* 45(6): 649-655.

Lan, C. C., G. S. Chen, et al. (2005). FK506 promotes melanocyte and melanoblast growth and creates a favourable milieu for cell migration via keratinocytes: possible mechanisms of how tacrolimus ointment induces repigmentation in patients with vitiligo. *Br J Dermatol* 153(3): 498-505.

Lapidoth, M., M. Adatto, et al. (2007). Targeted UVB phototherapy for psoriasis: a preliminary study. *Clin Exp Dermatol* 32(6): 642-645.

Larko, O. and G. Swanbeck (1982). Is UVB treatment of psoriasis safe? A study of extensively UVB-treated psoriasis patients compared with a matched control group. *Acta Derm Venereol* 62(6): 507-512.

Le Duff, F., E. Fontas, et al. (2010). 308-nm excimer lamp vs. 308-nm excimer laser for treating vitiligo: a randomized study. *Br J Dermatol* 163(1): 188-192.

Leone, G., P. Iacovelli, et al. (2003). Monochromatic excimer light 308 nm in the treatment of vitiligo: a pilot study. *J Eur Acad Dermatol Venereol* 17(5): 531-537.

Lim, J. L. and R. S. Stern (2005). High levels of ultraviolet B exposure increase the risk of non-melanoma skin cancer in psoralen and ultraviolet A-treated patients. *J Invest Dermatol* 124(3): 505-513.

Lotti, T., G. Buggiani, et al. (2008). Targeted and combination treatments for vitiligo. Comparative evaluation of different current modalities in 458 subjects. *Dermatol Ther* 21 Suppl 1: S20-26.

Lotti, T., L. Tripo, et al. (2009). Focused UV-B narrowband microphototherapy (Biopsorin). A new treatment for plaque psoriasis. *Dermatol Ther* 22(4): 383-385.

Lotti, T. M., G. Menchini, et al. (1999). UV-B radiation microphototherapy. An elective treatment for segmental vitiligo. *J Eur Acad Dermatol Venereol* 13(2): 102-108.

Lu-yan, T., F. Wen-wen, et al. (2006). Topical tacalcitol and 308-nm monochromatic excimer light: a synergistic combination for the treatment of vitiligo. *Photodermatol Photoimmunol Photomed* 22(6): 310-314.

Man, I., I. K. Crombie, et al. (2005). The photocarcinogenic risk of narrowband UVB (TL-01) phototherapy: early follow-up data. *Br J Dermatol* 152(4): 755-757.

Murase, J. E., E. E. Lee, et al. (2005). Effect of ethnicity on the risk of developing nonmelanoma skin cancer following long-term PUVA therapy. *Int J Dermatol* 44(12): 1016-1021.

Natta, R., T. Somsak, et al. (2003). Narrowband ultraviolet B radiation therapy for recalcitrant vitiligo in Asians. *J Am Acad Dermatol* 49(3): 473-476.

Nicolaidou, E., C. Antoniou, et al. (2007). Efficacy, predictors of response, and long-term follow-up in patients with vitiligo treated with narrowband UVB phototherapy. *J Am Acad Dermatol* 56(2): 274-278.

Nistico, S. P., R. Saraceno, et al. (2006). A 308-nm monochromatic excimer light in the treatment of palmoplantar psoriasis. *J Eur Acad Dermatol Venereol* 20(5): 523-526.

Njoo, M. D., J. D. Bos, et al. (2000). Treatment of generalized vitiligo in children with narrow-band (TL-01) UVB radiation therapy. *J Am Acad Dermatol* 42(2 Pt 1): 245-253.

Njoo, M. D. and W. Westerhof (2000). Guidelines for treatment of vitiligo: is an update pending If recommendations for children are not followed? *Arch Dermatol* 136(9): 1173-1174.

Noborio, R., K. Kobayashi, et al. (2006). Comparison of the efficacy of calcipotriol and maxacalcitol in combination with narrow-band ultraviolet B therapy for the treatment of psoriasis vulgaris. *Photodermatol Photoimmunol Photomed* 22(5): 262-264.

Nordal, E., G. Guleng, et al. (2011). Treatment of vitiligo with narrowband-UVB (TL01) combined with tacrolimus ointment (0.1%) vs. placebo ointment, a randomized right/left double-blind comparative study. *J Eur Acad Dermatol Venereol.*

Norris, D. A., T. Horikawa, et al. (1994). Melanocyte destruction and repopulation in vitiligo. *Pigment Cell Res* 7(4): 193-203.

Novak, Z., A. Berces, et al. (2004). Efficacy of different UV-emitting light sources in the induction of T-cell apoptosis. *Photochem Photobiol* 79(5): 434-439.

Novak, Z., B. Bonis, et al. (2002). Xenon chloride ultraviolet B laser is more effective in treating psoriasis and in inducing T cell apoptosis than narrow-band ultraviolet B. *J Photochem Photobiol B* 67(1): 32-38.

Ostovari, N., T. Passeron, et al. (2004). Treatment of vitiligo by 308-nm excimer laser: an evaluation of variables affecting treatment response. *Lasers Surg Med* 35(2): 152-156.

Ozawa, M., K. Ferenczi, et al. (1999). 312-nanometer ultraviolet B light (narrow-band UVB) induces apoptosis of T cells within psoriatic lesions. *J Exp Med* 189(4): 711-718.

Passeron, T., N. Ostovari, et al. (2004). Topical tacrolimus and the 308-nm excimer laser: a synergistic combination for the treatment of vitiligo. *Arch Dermatol* 140(9): 1065-1069.

Percivalle, S., R. Piccino, et al. (2008). Narrowband UVB phototherapy in vitiligo: evaluation of results in 53 patients. *G Ital Dermatol Venereol* 143(1): 9-14.

Pittelkow, M. R., H. O. Perry, et al. (1981). Skin cancer in patients with psoriasis treated with coal tar. A 25-year follow-up study. *Arch Dermatol* 117(8): 465-468.

Rath, N., H. K. Kar, et al. (2008). An open labeled, comparative clinical study on efficacy and tolerability of oral minipulse of steroid (OMP) alone, OMP with PUVA and broad / narrow band UVB phototherapy in progressive vitiligo. *Indian J Dermatol Venereol Leprol* 74(4): 357-360.

Roelandts, R. (2002). The history of phototherapy: something new under the sun? *J Am Acad Dermatol* 46(6): 926-930.

Samson Yashar, S., R. Gielczyk, et al. (2003). Narrow-band ultraviolet B treatment for vitiligo, pruritus, and inflammatory dermatoses. *Photodermatol Photoimmunol Photomed* 19(4): 164-168.

Saraceno, R., S. P. Nistico, et al. (2009). Monochromatic excimer light 308 nm in monotherapy and combined with topical khellin 4% in the treatment of vitiligo: a controlled study. *Dermatol Ther* 22(4): 391-394.

Sassi, F., S. Cazzaniga, et al. (2008). Randomized controlled trial comparing the effectiveness of 308-nm excimer laser alone or in combination with topical hydrocortisone 17-butyrate cream in the treatment of vitiligo of the face and neck. *Br J Dermatol* 159(5): 1186-1191.

Schallreuter, K. U. and H. Rokos (2007). From the bench to the bedside: proton pump inhibitors can worsen vitiligo. *Br J Dermatol* 156(6): 1371-1373.

Schulpis, C. H., C. Antoniou, et al. (1989). Phenylalanine plus ultraviolet light: preliminary report of a promising treatment for childhood vitiligo. *Pediatr Dermatol* 6(4): 332-335.

Shen, Z., T. W. Gao, et al. (2007). Optimal frequency of treatment with the 308-nm excimer laser for vitiligo on the face and neck. *Photomed Laser Surg* 25(5): 418-427.

Silverberg, N. B. (2010). Update on childhood vitiligo. *Curr Opin Pediatr* 22(4): 445-452.

Sitek, J. C., M. Loeb, et al. (2007). Narrowband UVB therapy for vitiligo: does the repigmentation last? *J Eur Acad Dermatol Venereol* 21(7): 891-896.

Spencer, J. M., R. Nossa, et al. (2002). Treatment of vitiligo with the 308-nm excimer laser: a pilot study. *J Am Acad Dermatol* 46(5): 727-731.

Stern, R. S. and N. Laird (1994). The carcinogenic risk of treatments for severe psoriasis. Photochemotherapy Follow-up Study. *Cancer* 73(11): 2759-2764.

Stinco, G., F. Piccirillo, et al. (2009). An open randomized study to compare narrow band UVB, topical pimecrolimus and topical tacrolimus in the treatment of vitiligo. *Eur J Dermatol* 19(6): 588-593.

Taneja, A., M. Trehan, et al. (2003). 308-nm excimer laser for the treatment of localized vitiligo. *Int J Dermatol* 42(8): 658-662.

Weichenthal, M. and T. Schwarz (2005). Phototherapy: how does UV work? *Photodermatol Photoimmunol Photomed* 21(5): 260-266.

Weischer, M., A. Blum, et al. (2004). No evidence for increased skin cancer risk in psoriasis patients treated with broadband or narrowband UVB phototherapy: a first retrospective study. *Acta Derm Venereol* 84(5): 370-374.

Westerhof, W. and L. Nieuweboer-Krobotova (1997). Treatment of vitiligo with UV-B radiation vs topical psoralen plus UV-A. *Arch Dermatol* 133(12): 1525-1528.

Wind, B. S., M. W. Kroon, et al. (2010). Home vs. outpatient narrowband ultraviolet B therapy for the treatment of nonsegmental vitiligo: a retrospective questionnaire study. *Br J Dermatol* 162(5): 1142-1144.

Wiskemann, A. (1978). [UVB-phototherapy of psoriasis using a standing box developed for PUVA-therapy]. *Z Hautkr* 53(18): 633-636.

Xiang, L. (2008). Once-weekly treatment of vitiligo with monochromatic excimer light 308 nm in Chinese patients. *J Eur Acad Dermatol Venereol* 22(7): 899-900.

Yang, Y. S., H. R. Cho, et al. (2010). Clinical study of repigmentation patterns with either narrow-band ultraviolet B (NBUVB) or 308 nm excimer laser treatment in Korean vitiligo patients. *Int J Dermatol* 49(3): 317-323.

Yones, S. S., R. A. Palmer, et al. (2007). Randomized double-blind trial of treatment of vitiligo: efficacy of psoralen-UV-A therapy vs Narrowband-UV-B therapy. *Arch Dermatol* 143(5): 578-584.

Zhang, X. Y., Y. L. He, et al. (2010). Clinical efficacy of a 308 nm excimer laser in the treatment of vitiligo. *Photodermatol Photoimmunol Photomed* 26(3): 138-142.

5

A Comparison of NB-UVB and PUVA in the Treatment of Vitiligo

Jiun-Yit Pan[1,2] and Robert P.E. Sarkany[2]
[1]National Skin Centre, Singapore
[2]St John's Institute of Dermatology, London
[1]Singapore
[2]UK

1. Introduction

Vitiligo is an acquired, progressive depigmenting disorder of the skin and mucous membranes in which melanocytes in affected skin are selectively destroyed. Theories regarding the mechanism of melanocyte destruction include autoimmune, cytotoxic, oxidative, and neural mechanisms. Vitiligo affects 0.5-2% of the world's population and the usual age of onset is in the third decade of life.

Photochemotherapy, along with phototherapy and topical therapy, are the most commonly utilized and effective vitiligo treatment modalities. Photochemotherapy for the treatment of vitiligo was historically used in ancient India and Egypt, where Hindus and Egyptians applied psoralen-containing plant extracts to depigmented vitiligo lesions where were then exposed to sunlight. These plants were found to be *Ammi majus* and *Psoralen corylefolia,* which contain 8-methoxypsoralen (8-MOP) and 5-methoxypsoralen (5-MOP).

Phototherapy has been shown in many studies to induce effective repigmentation in more than 70% of patients with early and/or localized disease. Narrow-band ultraviolet B radiation (NB-UVB) with an emission spectrum of 310-312 nanometers (nm) is a safe treatment modality that is often used two to three times weekly as monotherapy, or combined with topical steroids. The treatment is safe in children, pregnant women and lactating mothers, and has minimal adverse effects (xerosis, pruritus, skin aging, and tanning). The risk of skin cancer is minimal even with multiple treatments although there is a greater risk of phototoxicity with depigmented skin. NB-UVB has also been used in combination with antioxidants such as vitamin E.

Photochemotherapy involves the usage of psoralens combined with natural sunlight or UV light, usually ultraviolet A radiation (PUVA). 8-MOP or 5-MOP can be applied topically or used orally, followed by light exposure. Psoralens may not be used in pregnancy and there is a need for photoprotection following their use; there is as well a higher risk of burns, eye injury, and cutaneous malignancy than NB-UVB that may limit their cumulative usage. A 10-year retrospective study showed that PUVA is only moderately effective in widespread vitiligo (Kwok et al, 2002). Another small study from India successfully combined PUVA with a keratinocyte-melanocyte graft technique for stable vitiligo (Kachhawa et al, 2008).

Head-to-head comparison studies using NB-UVB and PUVA found both to be effective therapies - however, NB-UVB has been shown to induce even more stable repigmentation, is more convenient, and has fewer adverse effects when compared to PUVA.

2. Ultraviolet B phototherapy

Ultraviolet B (UVB) phototherapy is one of the most common vitiligo treatments used in the world today, and has evolved from the use of broadband ultraviolet B (BB-UVB) lamps to narrow-band ultraviolet B (NB-UVB) machines (Figure 1) with an emission spectrum of 310-315 nm (e.g. Philips TL-01). Vitiligo was the second most frequently treated disease by NB-UVB reported in a review published from a major U.S. phototherapy referral centre.

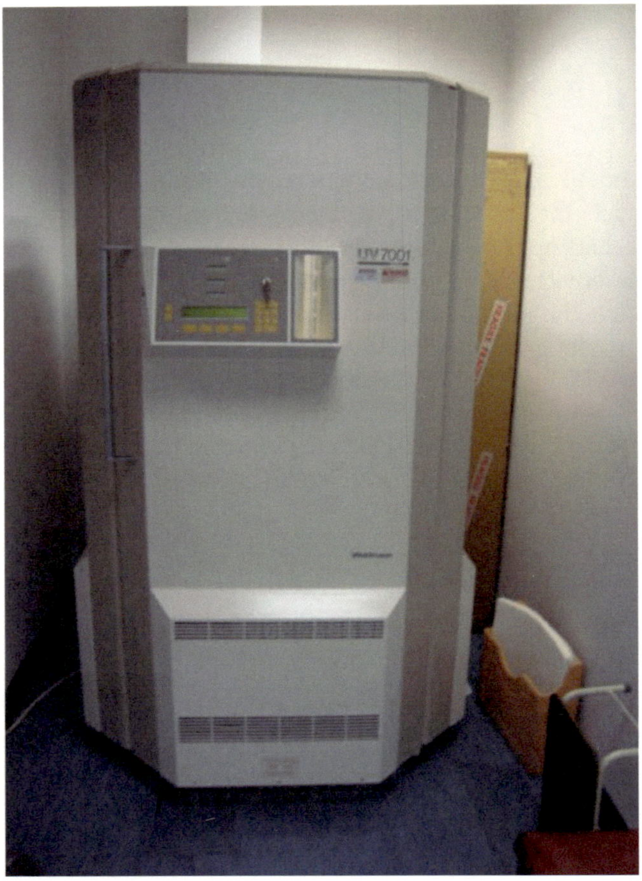

Fig. 1. A Narrowband UVB body box

UVB therapeutic modalities remain the mainstay of treatment for vitiligo due to its simplicity, safety and efficacy - a meta-analysis showed that it was the safest and most effective treatment for generalized vitiligo, with fewer adverse effects compared to psoralen and ultraviolet A (PUVA) therapy (Ngoo et al, 1996). Sixty-three studies were found on therapies for localized vitiligo. Among randomized controlled trials on localized vitiligo, the pooled odds ratio vs. placebo was significant for topical class 3 corticosteroids (14.32; 95%

confidence interval [CI], 2.45-83.72). Topical class 3 and class 4 corticosteroids carried the highest mean success rates (56% [95% CI, 50%-62%] and 55% [95% CI, 49%-61%], respectively). Side effects were reported mostly with topical psoralen and intralesional and class 4 corticosteroids. In randomized controlled trials on generalized vitiligo, the odds ratio vs. placebo was significant for oral methoxsalen plus sunlight (23.37; 95% CI, 1.33-409.93), oral psoralen plus sunlight (19.87; 95% CI, 2.37-166.32), and oral trioxsalen plus sunlight (3.75; 95% CI, 1.24-11.29). In this series, the highest mean success rates were achieved with NB-UVB (63%; 95% CI, 50%-76%), BB-UVB (57%; 95% CI, 29%-82%), and oral methoxsalen plus UVA therapy (51%; 95% CI, 46%-56%). Oral methoxsalen plus UVA was associated with the highest rates of side effects. No side effects were reported with UVB therapy.

Critical reviews and guidelines recommend that UVB light be the primary phototherapy option for vitiligo, especially for generalized disease. A retrospective study done at a major referral centre in the United States administered NB-UVB phototherapy as monotherapy three times a week (Scherschun et al, 2001). The starting dose was 280 mJ/cm^2, with 15% dose increments at each subsequent treatment. This treatment protocol resulted in rapid repigmentation in many patients, including those with skin phototypes IV and V.

Vitiliginous areas are considered to have a type 1 Fitzpatrick response to UV light. Treatments are usually 2-3 times weekly with initiation of dose at 50-70% of the average minimal erythema dose (MED) for NB-UVB treatment for type 1 skin (about 400 mJ/cm^2). The minimal erythema dose is the minimum dosage of UVB that produces just perceptible redness 24 hours after exposure. Patients should be referred to a dermatologist for UV radiation therapy. A total of 75 to 150 treatments (*e.g.* three times a week for 6 to 12 months) may be necessary. The course of therapy is usually much longer compared to inflammatory skin disorders such as atopic dermatitis and psoriasis, and the treatment course may last for years as long as there is continued gradual improvement and follicular repigmentation. However, the benefits of the usage of MED compared with fixed starting doses remains controversial. Fixed starting doses based on type 1 Fitzpatrick skin phototype allow an easier and more convenient means of initiating phototherapy, but do not take into account racial variations in MED. Also, many centres propose a lower maximum dose for NB-UVB in vitiligo compared to other inflammatory disorders (2 J/cm^2 for vitiligo compared to 5 J/cm^2 for psoriasis in our phototherapy unit).

NB-UVB has certain limitations. Lesions in acral sites are less likely to respond well to treatment than lesions on the face, trunk, or limbs. Segmental vitiligo is also less responsive to treatment. Long-standing lesions may also exhibit a lower rate of success in some cases.

Combination therapy with topical corticosteroids and NB-UVB is both effective and safe. NB-UVB has been used in combination with topical calcineurin inhibitors, and most studies show better improvement and repigmentation compared to NB-UVB monotherapy. Sixty-eight patients with vitiligo enrolled in a randomized, double-blind, placebo-controlled study (Esfandiarpour et al, 2009) in which patients were randomized into two groups: NB-UVB plus pimecrolimus or NB-UVB plus placebo, both for three months. NB-UVB three times a week was initiated at 280 mJ/cm^2, with 15% increments for each subsequent treatment until erythema was reported or a maximum of 800 mJ/cm^2 was achieved. At baseline, 6 weeks, and 12 weeks after commencement of therapy, vitiliginous patches were measured. No significant side effects were reported except self-limited erythema and pruritus. After 12 weeks of treatment, repigmentation of facial lesions was greater in patients treated with combined pimecrolimus and NB-UVB compared with the placebo plus NB-UVB group (64.3 vs. 25.1%, $p < 0.05$%). There was no statistically significant difference in the repigmentation rate between the two groups on other body areas. This study showed that on the face, NB-UVB works better if combined with pimecrolimus 1% cream rather than when used alone.

Another prospective single-blind study (Majid I 2010) was performed on 80 patients with generalized vitiligo over 12 years of age who had symmetrically distributed vitiligo lesions on the face, trunk or limbs. The patients applied topical tacrolimus 0.1% ointment twice daily on selected symmetrically distributed lesions on the left side of the body. No topical agent was applied on the corresponding lesions on the right. The patients also received whole-body NB-UVB exposure three times every week on non-consecutive days according to a set protocol. Lesions selected for the comparison analysis were photographed serially and assessed by a single-blinded observer for the extent of repigmentation achieved. The extent of repigmentation achieved was calculated on the basis of VASI (Vitiligo Area Scoring Index) scoring. The VASI score is a composite estimate of the overall area of vitiligo patches at baseline and the degree of macular repigmentation within these patches over time, ranging from 0-100%. The time taken until initial repigmentation, as well as overall repigmentation achieved, and adverse effects were noted and compared between corresponding lesions on each side. Seventy-four patients with 234 symmetrical vitiligo lesions were available for comparison analysis at the end of the study period. The mean repigmentation achieved on the left-sided study lesions was approximately 71% (VASI score of 4.0) as compared to 60.5% on the symmetrically distributed right-sided lesions (VASI score of 3.4). Moreover, the repigmentation started earlier on the lesions on left side than on the right-side. No significant adverse events were reported with combination treatment. In this study, addition of topical tacrolimus increased the extent of overall repigmentation achieved with NB-UVB therapy in vitiligo and also reduced the cumulative NB-UVB dose needed to achieve a therapeutic benefit in affected patients.

NB-UVB treatment was given to 24 patients with generalized vitiligo three times weekly in a study from Turkey (Goktas et al, 2006). Topical calcipotriol cream was only applied to the lesions located on the right side of the body and treatment was continued for 6 months. Treatment efficacy was evaluated by determining the average response rates of the lesions at 3-month intervals. The average response rates of patients receiving combination of NB-UVB plus calcipotriol and NB-UVB alone were 51 ±/- 19.6% and 39 ±/- 18.9%, respectively. The median cumulative UVB dose and number of UVB exposures for initial repigmentation were 6345 mJ/cm^2 (2,930-30,980 mJ/cm^2) and 18 mJ/cm^2 (12-67 mJ/cm^2) for the combination therapy, and 8867.5 mJ/cm^2 (2,500-30,980 mJ/cm^2) and 24 mJ/cm^2 (15-67 mJ/cm^2) for the NB-UVB therapy, respectively. These findings indicated that concurrent topical calcipotriol potentiates the efficacy of NB-UVB in the treatment of vitiligo. This combination not only provided earlier pigmentation with lower total UVB dosage and less adverse UVB effects, but also reduced the duration and cost of treatment.

3. Psoralen with ultraviolet A (PUVA) therapy

Vitiligo was the first described indication for psoralen with ultraviolet A (PUVA) treatment (Parrish et al, 1976) PUVA (Figure 2) is less used now since NB-UVB has been described as a safe and effective alternative (Bhatnagar et al, 2007). Psoralens are phototoxic compounds that interact with various components of cells and absorb photons to produce photochemical reactions altering the function of cellular constituents - they may be consumed orally or applied topically to the skin, in combination with long-wave ultraviolet A (UVA) radiation. For topical application, the patient may bathe in a dilute methoxsalen solution or have the solution directly applied to affected areas. Psoralens may not be used in pregnancy and there is a higher risk of burns, cutaneous malignancy and eye injury.

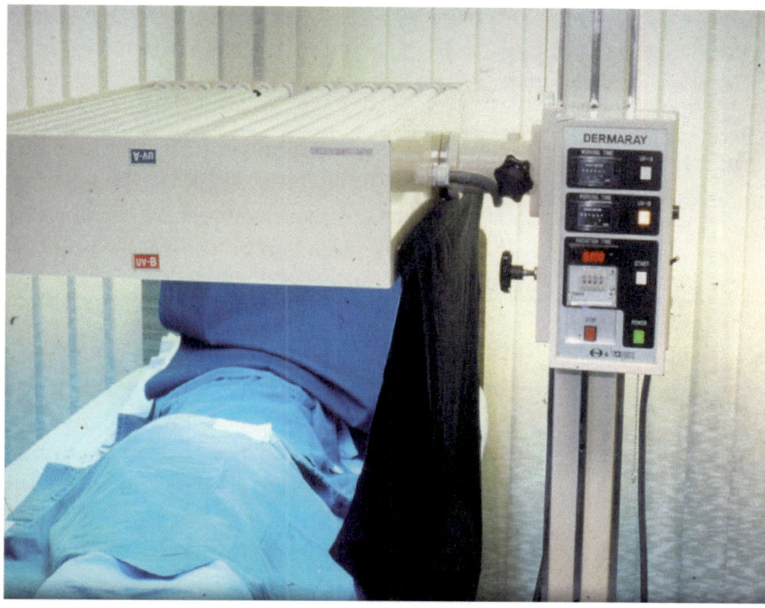

Fig. 2. A targeted UVA light source for PUVA therapy

Patients are treated as Fitzpatrick skin type I individuals and the therapeutic objective is to maintain minimal light pink reactions in patches of depigmented skin. About 100-200 exposures are required to produce maximal repigmentation and about 70% of patients respond. Sessions are usually 2-3 times weekly. Guidelines for psoralen administration and PUVA protocols for vitiligo are suggested below in Table 1 and Table 2. A comparison of PUVA and NBUVB for the treatment of vitiligo can be found in Table 3.

Concurrent use of topical corticosteroids has been shown to enhance the response to PUVA therapy. There have been a number of recent publications combining topical vitamin D analogues with PUVA therapy which show a beneficial synergistic effect, but more studies are required.

A placebo-controlled double-blind study (Ermis et al, 2001) was done in Turkey to investigate whether the effectiveness of PUVA treatment could be enhanced by combination with topical calcipotriol. Thirty-five patients with generalized vitiligo enrolled in the study. Symmetrical lesions of similar dimensions and with no spontaneous repigmentation on arms, legs or trunk were selected as reference lesions. In this randomized left-right comparison study, calcipotriol cream or placebo was applied to the reference lesions an hour before PUVA treatment (oral 8-MOP and conventional UVA units) twice weekly. Patients were examined at weekly intervals. The mean number of sessions and the cumulative UVA dosage for initial and complete repigmentation were calculated for twenty-seven patients. The mean cumulative UVA dose and number of UVA exposures for initial repigmentation were 52.52 ± 6.10 J/cm^2 and 9.33 ± 0.65 on the calcipotriol side, and 78.20 ± 7.88 J/cm^2 and 12.00 ± 0.81 on the placebo side, respectively ($P < 0.001$). For complete repigmentation, respective values were 232.79 ± 14.97 J/cm^2 and 27.40 ± 1.47 on the calcipotriol side and 259.93 ± 13.71 J/cm^2 and 30.07 ± 1.34 on the placebo side (P = 0.001). Treatment with calcipotriol and PUVA resulted in significantly higher percentages of repigmentation for both initial (81%) and complete pigmentation (63%), compared with placebo and PUVA (7% and 15%, respectively). These results showed that concurrent topical calcipotriol potentiates the efficacy of PUVA in the treatment of vitiligo, and that this combination achieved earlier pigmentation with a lower total UVA dosage.

Oral 8-Methoxypsoralen (8-MOP)	8-MOP is taken 2 hours before treatment, at a dose of 25 mg/m^2 (Ibbotson et al 2001). The body surface area is calculated using a normogram. Basing the dose on body surface area is preferable to basing the dose only on body weight.
Oral 5-Methoxypsoralen (5-MOP)	5-MOP is taken 3 hours before treatment at a dose of 50 mg/m^2.
Bath PUVA (Halpern et al 2000)	30 mls of 8-MOP 1.2% solution is added to 100 mls of water (=3.6 mg/L at 37 °C), and the patient is immersed for 15 minutes. UVA exposure is given immediately. Patients do not need to shower afterwards but should have sunscreen applied to any areas that will be exposed to sunshine in the next 4 hours.
Hand-Foot Immersion PUVA (Halpern et al 2000)	1.3 mls of 8-MOP 1.2% solution is added to 4 litres of water (3.9 mg/L at 37 °C) and the patient's hands or feet are immersed for 15 minutes. UVA exposure is ideally given 30 minutes afterwards but can be given immediately. The hands / feet need not be washed afterwards, but should have sunscreen applied if they will be subsequently exposed to sunshine in the next few hours.
Gel PUVA (Halpern et al 2000)	A thin layer of 0.005% gel is applied to the diseased area using a gloved hand. UVA exposure is given 30 minutes later.

Table 1. Psoralen Administration

Psoralen and solar ultraviolet A (PUVAsol) involves the exposure of the patient to sunlight after administration of oral or topical psoralen. A study (Pathak et al 1984) compared different psoralen compounds, doses and combinations, combined with exposure to sunlight. There was considerable regional variation in response, with the face showing the best response and the acral areas the worst response. Approximately 45% of participants treated with the combination of 8-methoxypsoralen (8-MOP) and trimethylpsoralen (TMP) achieved full repigmentation of the head and nearly 60% achieved 75 to 100% repigmentation of the head and neck, which was statistically significant when compared to placebo. However, 49% of all participants reported side effects including nausea, pruritus, dizziness, headaches, eye discomfort and gastrointestinal symptoms, with the rate of complications highest in the group which used 8-MOP and TMP in combination. Khalid et al (1995) showed that clobetasol propionate was significantly better than PUVASOL at achieving at least 75% repigmentation in vitiligo patients (RR 4.70 95%CI 1.14 to 19.39).

Siddiqui et al (1994) examined the effectiveness of a combination of oral L-phenylalanine (L-Phe) and UVA in an open trial and a small double-blind trial, which showed equivocal results. Phenylalanine is an amino acid that is the precursor of tyrosine, which is required for melanin pigment synthesis. Oral L-Phe loading resulted in peak plasma levels of L-Phe after 30-60 minutes and a slight increase in the plasma tyrosine level. Response to L-Phe plus UVA irradiation was positive, and various grades of repigmentation not exceeding 77% in the open and 60% in the blind trial were observed. An increased L-Phe dose resulted in increased L-Phe plasma levels but not in improved clinical results. The optimal L-Phe dose appeared to be lower than 50 milligrams/kilograms/day.

	Frequency of Treatment	Initial Dose	Incremental Doses	Maximum single dose
Oral PUVA	Twice a week	0.5 J/cm^2	0.25 J/cm^2 increase at each visit until maximum dose reached. If erythema develops, omit treatment until settled and reduce to the previous dose, then use increments of 0.1-0.25 J/cm^2 if no erythema	5 J/cm^2
Bath PUVA	Twice a week	0.05 J/cm^2 to face 0.1 J/cm^2 to other sites	0.05 J/cm^2 increase at each visit until maximum dose reached. If erythema develops, omit treatment until settled and reduce to the previous dose, then use increments of 0.02-0.05 J/cm^2 if no erythema	1 J/cm^2
Gel PUVA	Twice a week	0.5 J/cm^2	0.25 J/cm^2 increase at each visit until maximum dose reached. If erythema develops, omit treatment until settled and reduce to the previous dose, then use increments of 0.1-0.25 J/cm^2 if no erythema	1 J/cm^2

Table 2. PUVA protocols for vitiligo

Camacho et al (2002) conducted an open trial on 70 patients with active vitiligo, where they were treated with oral and topical phenylalanine, clobetasol cream at night, sunlight in the spring and summer and UVA phototherapy in autumn and winter. Nearly 69% of patients achieved an improvement of 75% or more, but the improvement was only modest in patients with focal and segmental vitiligo.

PUVA has also been combined effectively with a keratinocyte-melanocyte graft technique for stable vitiligo in a study from India (Kachhawa et al 2008). This autologous, non-cultured, non-trypsinized, melanocyte plus keratinocyte grafting technique is a new and simple method of vitiligo surgery. In the trial, eighteen vitiligo patches underwent this procedure. The upper layer of epidermis was removed by superficial dermabrasion using a dermabrader micromotor until the epidermis appeared wet and shiny. Then, antibiotic ointment was applied and dermabrasion was continued until the whitish area of the upper dermis was apparent. The paste-like material (ointment with entangled epidermal particles) was collected and spread over the dermabraded recipient site. Pigmentation usually started at 4-6 weeks, and then PUVA therapy was initiated. Complete uniform pigmentation took 16-20 weeks. For smaller vitiligo patches this method gives cosmetically acceptable results. It is fairly easy to perform and does not require specific laboratory setup.

	NB-UVB	PUVA
Ease of Administration	Simple, no prior preparation required	Requires topical / bath application or consumption of psoralen. PUVASOL allows patient to apply topical meladinine paint at home, followed by self-exposure to ambient sunlight.
Targeted therapy available for localized vitiligo?	Yes (Multiclear, Excimer lamp etc)	Yes
Efficacy	Both are equally effective for vitiligo. Acral and periorificial areas are more resistant to phototherapy. A meta-analysis (Ngoo et al, 1996) showed that NB-UVB is the safest and most effective treatment for generalized vitiligo, with fewer adverse effects compared to psoralen and ultraviolet A (PUVA) therapy.	
Adverse Effects	Sunburn, itch, tanning and skin ageing. Safe in pregnancy.	Adverse effects related to photosensitivity from psoralen administration – need for sun protection and sun avoidance, including eye protection for oral PUVA (risk of cataracts). Oral PUVA can cause nausea and vomiting and its safety has not been established during pregnancy.
Long-term safety	Minimal skin cancer risk even with multiple treatments.	Increased risk of non-melanoma skin cancer and melanoma with prolonged treatment, especially in Caucasian skin.

Table 3. Comparison between NB-UVB and PUVA

There has been a concern regarding the potential carcinogenicity of prolonged PUVA therapy, especially the increased incidence of non-melanoma skin cancer and malignant melanoma. Information from 4799 Swedish patients (2343 men, 2456 women) who had received PUVA between 1974 and 1985 was linked to the compulsory Swedish Cancer Registry in order to identify individuals with cancer (Lindelöf B et al 1999). The average follow-up period was 15.9 years for men and 16.2 for women. The authors did not find any increased risk for malignant melanoma in their total cohort of 4799 patients treated with PUVA or in a subcohort comprising 1867 patients followed for 15-21 years. For cutaneous SCC there was an increase in the risk: the relative risk was 5.6 (95% confidence interval, CI 4. 4-7.1) for men and 3.6 (95% CI 2.1-5.8) for women.
However, the majority of research demonstrating an increased incidence of skin cancer with psoralen plus ultraviolet A (PUVA) therapy had mainly reflected the Caucasian experience. A study (Murase JE et al 2005) was done of 4,294 long-term PUVA patients in Japan, Korea, Thailand, Egypt, and Tunisia with a follow-up period of at least 5 years. The relative risk of PUVA patients developing non-melanoma skin cancer relative to general dermatology outpatients was 0.86 [CI 0.36-1.35]. The study showed that there does not appear to be an increased risk of nonmelanoma skin cancer with long-term PUVA therapy in Asian and Arabian-African populations. Thus, in phototherapy risk assessment, it is important to consider the patient's skin phototype and the potential protection that more pigmented skin may confer.

4. Guidance from the British Association of Dermatologists guidelines and the Cochrane review

The British Association of Dermatologists (BAD) published clinical guidelines on the management of vitiligo (2008) that recommend that NB-UVB phototherapy (or PUVA) should be considered only in patients who cannot be adequately managed with conservative topical treatments, have widespread disease, or have localized disease significantly impacting quality of life.
For non-segmental vitiligo, NB-UVB is preferred to PUVA because of greater efficacy. The BAD also recommends an arbitrary limit of 200 treatments with NBUVB for patients with skin types I–III, and 150 treatments with PUVA for patients with skin types I–III. This is in view of the greater susceptibility of depigmented skin to sunburn and photodamage due to absence of melanin.
A Cochrane review on the management of vitiligo (2006, updated in 2010) showed limited-to-moderate evidence for various types and regimens of phototherapy (UVA and UVB) used alone or in combination with psoralens, calcipotriol, folic acid and vitamin B12, oral L-phenylalanine and topical pseudocatalase. Topical khellin combined with UVA is commonly used throughout the world but there is a lack of evidence of its benefit. This is also the case for topical tacrolimus and topical calcipotriol used in conjunction with ultraviolet light, oral Ginkgo biloba, and thin split-thickness grafts. The reviewers recommended that more randomized controlled trials are needed to fully establish the efficacy and safety of widely used interventions such as steroids, photochemotherapy using PUVA or khellin and NB-UVB monotherapy. In the future, these should also incorporate patient-centred outcomes such as quality of life indices.

5. Conclusion

Conventional therapies for vitiligo require months to years of treatment and sometimes result in disappointing outcomes, particularly in difficult areas in the extremities. Thus far, NBUVB has remained as one of the most effective and safe treatments for vitiligo and the options of targeted phototherapy and combinations with various topical modalities provide additional choices in the dermatologist's armamentarium. PUVA therapy has also been clearly shown to be efficacious but is associated with a higher risk of the adverse effects due to psoralen administration, and an increased risk of skin cancer especially in Caucasian skin.

6. References

[1] CL Hexsel, RH Huggins, HW Lim. Light-Based Therapies for Skin of Color 2009, 171-187, DOI: 10.1007/978-1-84882-328-0_6.

[2] Matz H, Tur E. Vitiligo. Curr Probl Dermatol. 2007;35:78-102.

[3] Yashar SS, Gielczyk R, Scherschun L, Lim HW. Narrow-band ultraviolet B for vitiligo, pruritus, and inflammatory dermatoses. Photodermatol Photoimmunol Photomed 2003; 19: 164–168.

[4] Njoo MD, Spuls PI, Bos JD, Westerhof W, Bossuyt MM. Nonsurgical repigmentation therapies in vitiligo. Metaanalysis of the literature. Arch Dermatol 1998;134:1532-40.

[5] Asawanonda P, Charoenlap M, Korkij W. Treatment of localized vitiligo with targeted broadband UVB phototherapy: A pilot study. Photodermatol Photoimmunol Photomed 2006;22:133-6

[6] Pravit Asawanonda, Jirasin Kijluakiat , Wiwat Korkij and Wannasri Sindhupak. Targeted Broadband Ultraviolet B Phototherapy Produces Similar Responses to Targeted Narrowband Ultraviolet B Phototherapy for Vitiligo: A Randomized, Double-blind Study. Acta Derm Venereol 2008; 88: 376–381

[7] Njoo MD, Westerhof W, Bos JD, Bossuyt PM. The development of guidelines for the treatment of vitiligo. Clinical Epidemiology Unit of the Istituto Dermopatico dell'Immacolata-Istituto di Recovero e Cura a Carattere Scientifico (IDI-IRCCS) and the Archives of Dermatology. Arch Dermatol 1999; 135:1514.

[8] Scherschun L, Kim JJ, Lim HW. Narrow-band ultraviolet B is a useful and well-tolerated treatment for vitiligo. J Am Acad Dermatol 2001; 44:999.

[9] Anbar TS, Westerhof W, Abdel-Rahman AT, El-Khayyat MA. Evaluation of the effects of NB-UVB in both segmental and non-segmental vitiligo affecting different body sites. Photodermatol Photoimmunol Photomed 2006; 22:157.

[10] Brazzelli V, Antoninetti M, Palazzini S, et al. Critical evaluation of the variants influencing the clinical response of vitiligo: study of 60 cases treated with ultraviolet B narrow-band phototherapy. J Eur Acad Dermatol Venereol 2007; 21:1369.

[11] Esfandiarpour I, Ekhlasi A, Farajzadeh S, Shamsadini S. The efficacy of pimecrolimus 1% cream plus narrow-band ultraviolet B in the treatment of vitiligo: a double-blind, placebo-controlled clinical trial. J Dermatolog Treat 2009; 20:14.

[12] Mehrabi D, Pandya AG. A randomized, placebo-controlled, double-blind trial comparing narrowband UV-B Plus 0.1% tacrolimus ointment with narrowband UV-B plus placebo in the treatment of generalized vitiligo. Arch Dermatol 2006; 142:927.

[13] Majid I. Does topical tacrolimus ointment enhance the efficacy of narrowband ultraviolet B therapy in vitiligo? A left-right comparison study. Photodermatol Photoimmunol Photomed 2010; 26:230.

[14] Sassi F, Cazzaniga S, Tessari G, et al. Randomized controlled trial comparing the effectiveness of 308-nm excimer laser alone or in combination with topical hydrocortisone 17-butyrate cream in the treatment of vitiligo of the face and neck. Br J Dermatol 2008; 159:1186.

[15] Passeron T, Ostovari N, Zakaria W, et al. Topical tacrolimus and the 308-nm excimer laser: a synergistic combination for the treatment of vitiligo. Arch Dermatol 2004; 140:1065.

[16] Lu-yan T, Wen-wen F, Lei-hong X, et al. Topical tacalcitol and 308-nm monochromatic excimer light: a synergistic combination for the treatment of vitiligo. Photodermatol Photoimmunol Photomed 2006; 22:310.

[17] Goktas EO, Aydin F, Senturk N, et al. Combination of narrow band UVB and topical calcipotriol for the treatment of vitiligo. J Eur Acad Dermatol Venereol 2006; 20:553.

[18] Tjioe M, Gerritsen MJ, Juhlin L, van de Kerkhof PC. Treatment of vitiligo vulgaris with narrow band UVB (311 nm) for one year and the effect of addition of folic acid and vitamin B12. Acta Derm Venereol. 2002;82(5):369-72.

[19] Parrish JA, Fitzpatrick TB, Shea C, et al. Photochemotherapy of vitiligo. Arch Dermatol 1976;112:1531-4.

[20] Lassus A, Halme K, Eskelinen A, et al. Treatment of vitiligo with oral methoxsalen and UVA. Photodermatology 1984:1:170-3.

[21] Pathak MA, Mosher DB, Fitzpatrick TB, et al. Safety and therapeutic effectiveness of 8-methoxypsoralen, 4,5,8-trimethylpsoralen, and psoralen in vitiligo. Natl Cancer Inst Monogr 1984;66:165-73.

[22] Bhatnagar A, Kanwar AJ, Parsad D. Comparison of systemic PUVA and NB-UVB in the treatment of vitiligo: an open prospective study. J Eur Acad Dermatol Venereol 2007; 21:638–42.

[23] Grimes PE, Minus HR, Chakrabarti SG, Enterline J, Halder R, Gough JE, Kenney JA Jr. Determination of optimal topical photochemotherapy for vitiligo. J Am Acad Dermatol. 1982 Dec;7(6):771-8.

[24] Ermis O, Alpsoy E, Cetin L, Yilmaz E. Is the efficacy of psoralen plus ultraviolet A therapy for vitiligo enhanced by concurrent topical calcipotriol? A placebo-controlled double-blind study. Br J Dermatol 2001; 145:472.

[25] Parsad D, Saini R, Verma N. Combination of PUVAsol and topical calcipotriol in vitiligo. Dermatology 1998; 197:167.

[26] Khalid M, Mujtaba G, Haroon TS. Comparison of 0.05% clobetasol propionate cream and topical Puvasol in childhood vitiligo. Int J Dermatol. 1995 Mar;34(3):203-5

[27] Siddiqui AH, Stolk LM, Bhaggoe R, Hu R, Schutgens RB, Westerhof W. L-phenylalanine and UVA irradiation in the treatment of vitiligo. Dermatology. 1994;188(3):215-8

[28] Camacho F, Mazuecos J. Oral and topical L-phenylalanine, clobetasol propionate, and UVA/sunlight--a new study for the treatment of vitiligo. J Drugs Dermatol. 2002 Sep;1(2):127-31

[29] Kachhawa D, Kalla G. Keratinocyte-melanocyte graft technique followed by PUVA therapy for stable vitiligo. Indian J Dermatol Venereol Leprol. 2008 Nov-Dec;74(6):622-4.

[30] Lindelöf B, Sigurgeirsson B, Tegner E, Larkö O, Johannesson A, Berne B, Ljunggren B, Andersson T, Molin L, Nylander-Lundqvist E, Emtestam L. PUVA and cancer risk: the Swedish follow-up study. Br J Dermatol. 1999 Jul;141(1):108-12.
[31] Murase JE, Lee EE, Koo J. Effect of ethnicity on the risk of developing nonmelanoma skin cancer following long-term PUVA therapy. Int J Dermatol. 2005 Dec;44(12):1016-21.
[32] Gawkrodger DJ, Ormerod AD, Shaw L, Mauri-Sole I, Whitton ME, Watts MJ, Anstey AV, Ingham J, Young K; Therapy Guidelines and Audit Subcommittee, British Association of Dermatologists; Clinical Standards Department, Royal College of Physicians of London; Cochrane Skin Group; Vitiligo Society. Guideline for the diagnosis and management of vitiligo. Br J Dermatol. 2008 Nov;159(5):1051-76.
[33] Whitton ME, Ashcroft DM, Barrett CW, Gonzalez U. Interventions for vitiligo. Cochrane Database Syst Rev. 2006 Jan 25;(1):CD003263.
[34] Whitton ME, Pinart M, Batchelor J, Lushey C, Leonardi-Bee J, González U. Interventions for vitiligo. Cochrane Database Syst Rev. 2010 Jan 20;(1):CD003263.
[35] Halpern SM, Anstey AV, Dawe RS, Diffey BL, Farr PM, Ferguson J, Hawk JL, Ibbotson S, McGregor JM, Murphy GM, Thomas SE, Rhodes LE. Guidelines for topical PUVA: a report of a workshop of the British photodermatology group. Br J Dermatol. 2000 Jan;142(1):22-31.
[36] Ibbotson SH, Dawe RS, Farr PM. The effect of methoxsalen dose on ultraviolet-A-induced erythema. J Invest Dermatol. 2001 May;116(5):813-5.

6

Systemic Corticosteroids in Vitiligo

Binod K. Khaitan and Sushruta Kathuria
Department of Dermatology and Venereology
All India Institute of Medical Sciences, New Delhi
India

1. Introduction

Vitiligo is an acquired disorder characterized by depigmented macules on skin, hair, and mucosa. Its prevalence worldwide is 0.1-2% and varies from country to country.[1] It is associated with high psychiatric morbidity and dysfunction, particularly in darker skin types where the contrast between normal and depigmented skin is highly pronounced.[2,3] The usual approach to the treatment of vitiligo has been to regain pigment in vitiliginous areas rather than controlling the disease process. This is akin to treating the *effects* of the disease rather than treating the disease itself. Such an approach frequently results in frustration because patients can continue to develop new lesions at other sites even while existing lesions are repigmenting, or the disease may be reactivated at a later stage even after achieving a fair degree of therapeutic success.[4] Therefore, the important priority for the treatment of vitiligo should be first to control the disease process, and then taking measures to repigment existing lesions.

Systemic corticosteroids are a broad group of drugs that are widely used in various dermatological and non-dermatological conditions. Corticosteroids, both topical and systemic, have been used in vitiligo for over four decades with some concern about its efficacy as well as its known or expected adverse effects. Further research may provide evidence that systemic corticosteroids may be an important modality for the treatment of progressive vitiligo.

2. History

In 1967, oral corticosteroids were used for the first time in vitiligo. Triamcinolone orally was found to have a synergistic effect with methoxypsoralen as compared to methoxypsoralen alone.[5] In 1976, adrenocorticotropic hormone (ACTH) was found to be effective in inducing repigmentation in patients who had previously failed photochemotherapy with psoralen followed by UVA exposure (PUVA).[6] In the same year, a mixture of prednisolone, betamethasone, paramethasone acetate and methylprednisolone given orally was effective in producing satisfactory repigmentation in one-third of patients studied, thus confirming the efficacy of corticosteroids in vitiligo.[7] Treatment of vitiligo is known to be long-term, hence the question of long term safety of systemic corticosteroids is an important consideration. To reduce long-term complications of corticosteroids, oral mini-pulse therapy was introduced in 1989 and was established in 1993, where instead of daily oral corticosteroids, a long-acting corticosteroid was given on two consecutive days of the week.[8,9] Since then, systemic corticosteroids are used in day-to-day practice in extensive and progressive vitiligo.

3. Structure and classification

The structure of corticosteroids consists of three hexane rings and one pentane ring known as the cyclopentanoperhydrophenathrene nucleus. The different systemic corticosteroids are variations of this basic structure. Systemic corticosteroids are classified according to their half-lives. (Table 1)

Corticosteroid	Equivalent dose (mg)	Glucocorticoid potency	Mineralocorticoid potency	Plasma half- life (minutes)	Biological half-life (hours)
Short Acting					
Cortisone	25	0.8	2+	30-90	8-12
Hydrocortisone	20	1	2+	60-120	8-12
Deflazacort	6			90-120	<12
Intermediate Acting					
Prednisone	5	4	1+	60	24-36
Prednisolone	5	4	1+	115-212	24-36
Methylprednisolone	4	5	0	180	24-36
Triamcinolone	4	5	0	78-188	24-36
Long Acting					
Dexamethasone	0.75	20-30	0	100-300	36-54
Betamethasone	0.6-0.75	20-30	0	100-300	36-54

Table 1. Classification of Corticosteroids[10,11]

The structure, mechanism of action, and pharmacokinetic profile of various systemic corticosteroids are similar. The main difference is in their glucocorticoid and mineralocorticoid effects and biological half-life. Hence, the choice of corticosteroid is decided by the duration of action needed, the dosing schedule to be used (daily versus weekly) and the clinical profile of the patient. Having a working knowledge of equivalent dosing helps in dose conversion when one corticosteroid is switched to another.

4. Mechanism of action of corticosteroids in vitiligo

Vitiligo is considered to be primarily an autoimmune condition that results in the loss of melanocytes. Melanocytes are lost in vitiligo due to the destruction of melanocytes by humoral or intrinsic cellular mechanisms.[12] Humoral mechanisms involve destruction of melanocytes by pathogenic autoantibodies directed against melanocytes and the tyrosinase enzyme. Cellular mechanisms are as important as humoral in destroying melanocytes. Biopsies from vitiligo lesions show mild mononuclear infiltrate in the margins of lesional skin in active vitiligo with or without basal vacuolization. Active lesions show increased numbers of CD4+ T cells and increased epidermal expression of ICAM-1.[13] Peripheral T-cell activation is also seen in nonsegmental vitiligo and T-cell dysregulation is not only limited to the lesions.[14] The peripheral blood of vitiligo patients express more of the cutaneous lymphocyte-associated antigen positive melanocyte-specific cytotoxic T lymphocytes indicating that there is recruitment of T cells in the circulation to the skin.[15] Both the CD4+ and CD8+ T cells from perilesional and non-lesional skin in vitiligo show polarization towards the Type 1 cytokine profile which parallels depigmentation.[16] The melanocyte-specific cytotoxic T cells found in perilesional biopsies have the ability to infiltrate normal skin and destroy the melanocytes.[17] Besides cytotoxic T cells, regulatory T cells (T regs) also have a role in vitiligo. The T reg population is not decreased in the peripheral circulation, however, these T regs are not able to settle in the skin and this defect seems to be crucial in the observed perpetual anti-melanocyte reactivity in progressive disease.[18]

Corticosteroids suppress autoantibody formation and likely induce apoptosis of cytotoxic T cells. The autoimmune hypothesis still prevails in the pathogenesis of non-segmental vitiligo, and the autoimmune process is not limited to the skin. In progressive disease, there is continuous assault on melanocytes. Topical corticosteroids, tacrolimus or any other topical agent may suppress autoimmune dysfunction at the site of a vitiligo lesion, but these do not have any effect on the disease process per se. Photochemotherapy and phototherapy stimulate melanocytes to cause repigmentation and have minimal immunomodulatory action on T-lymphocytes, but may not halt the rapid destruction of melanocytes. Systemic corticosteroids act not only on lesional immune activity, but also on the T cells in peripheral circulation. Besides modulating cell-mediated immunity, corticosteroids also suppress autoantibody formation. The serum of actively spreading vitiligo patients who received oral corticosteroids and showed improvement had a decrease in complement-mediated cytotoxicity by melanocyte autoantibodies and a reduced antibody titer to the melanocyte surface antigen.[19]

5. Indications

Systemic corticosteroids are the first-line treatment when a patient presents with rapidly progressive vitiligo. It helps not only in halting progression of the disease but also induces repigmentation as normal melanocytes from the periphery of the lesions or perifollicular area take over, once the process of melanocyte destruction is arrested. Assessment of treatment response is important and since the patient is not always sure whether new lesions have appeared or not since corticosteroid initiation, a baseline photographic record must be taken before starting treatment and periodically throughout treatment, preferably at 4-week intervals. The time taken for disease activity to stop is variable and may range from a few weeks to months. Once stability is achieved (defined as no new lesion formation and no extension of existing lesions), one must taper the corticosteroids slowly and add other modalities for augmentation of repigmentation.

Patients with extensive slowly progressive vitiligo (body surface area more than 10% with the continuous appearance of new lesions or slow extension of existing lesions) may also benefit from systemic corticosteroids as this suggests "simmering" autoimmune activity that may be long-term. Besides maintenance therapy, episodic treatment for 8-12 weeks at a time can also be added whenever there is relapse.

For example, systemic corticosteroids can also be added to photochemotherapy or phototherapy when there is transient fluctuation or worsening of disease activity. It can also be an adjuvant to surgery in both segmental and nonsegmental vitiligo.[20,21]

It is not advisable to use corticosteroid monotherapy in segmental vitiligo because segmental vitiligo is known to stabilize after some time. The initial period of progression may be rapid in segmental vitiligo, but nearly all lesions stabilize and remain confined to one part of the body. Hence use of corticosteroids may not be advisable. Patients with stable vitiligo will also not benefit from corticosteroids because they are not simply repigmentation agents; rather their efficacy comes from their effects on active disease. Universal or near-universal vitiligo is also not an indication for the use of corticosteroids since treatment is usually depigmentation of residual pigmented areas.

6. Modes of administration

Systemic corticosteroids given orally are effective in halting progression of vitiligo and producing repigmentation. However, the long treatment duration required in vitiligo raises concern about the long-term cumulative side effects of corticosteroids. Daily doses or alternate day dosing is thereby avoided in vitiligo. Therefore, oral mini pulse therapy (OMP) is preferred for the planned long-term maintenance therapy for 6 months or beyond.[9] OMP refers to giving a higher than the usual daily dose of corticosteroid on two consecutive days a week and leaving the remaining five days treatment-free. A long-acting corticosteroid is preferred so that the effect lasts for about 3 days at a time. Corticotropin and cortisol levels fall rapidly after the second dose of drug, but returns to baseline before the next dexamethasone pulse.[22] Hence, it is preferred to give a long-acting corticosteroid on two consecutive days in a week rather than once in three days to give the hypothalamic-pituitary-adrenal axis (HPA) axis time to revert back to normal before the next dose. The standard regimen is to give oral betamethasone 5 mg (5 of the 1 mg betamethasone tablets) after breakfast on Saturday and Sunday (or any other two consecutive days) every week.[9] Dexamethasone pulse has been used in doses of 5 mg or 10 mg in this manner.[22,23] Betamethasone pulse has been given as an adjunct with surgery.[24] Besides this standard regimen, there can be variations in OMP. If no response is seen, the dose can be increased from 5 mg upto 7.5 mg. In children, dose is reduced from 5 mg to 2.5-4 mg. Additional immunosuppressants, for example, cyclophosphamide and azathioprine, may also be added to the therapeutic regimen.

Methylprednisolone[25] has been used intravenously as high dose pulse therapy given on 3 consecutive days in a month but should not be considered as first-line treatment. Daily low dose prednisolone has also been used in tapering doses to discontinuation.[26,27]

The intramuscular route is not preferred as it is painful, and the level of drug in the circulation is unpredictable and good results are achieved by oral administration.

Monitoring of weight, fasting blood sugar, and blood pressure every month is necessary for any patient on systemic corticosteroids. Baseline and periodic photographs should also be done to monitor treatment response and repigmentation.

7. Side effects and contraindications

Systemic corticosteroids are known to have a variety of adverse effects. The predominant side effects are described in Table 2. However, these adverse effects do depend on dose, duration of treatment, and individual susceptibility. All patients do not develop the same adverse effects. Therefore, clinical evaluation and monitoring is the best way to ascertain whether adverse effects are minimal or serious, and reversible or irreversible. Minimal and reversible side effects are acceptable for continuing treatment.

System Affected	Side Effects
HPA Axis	Steroid withdrawal syndrome, Addisonian crisis
Metabolic	Hyperglycemia, increased appetite and weight gain, hypertension, congestive heart failure, hypokalemia, hypertriglyceridemia, cushingoid changes, menstrual irregularities
Bone	Osteoporosis, osteonecrosis, hypocalcemia
Gastrointestinal	Peptic ulcer disease, bowel perforation, fatty liver changes, esophageal reflux, nausea, vomiting
Ocular	Cataracts, glaucoma, infections
Psychiatric	Psychosis, agitation, depression
Neurological	Pseudotumor cerebri, peripheral neuropathy
Muscular	Myopathy
Cutaneous	Delayed wound healing, acneiform eruption, purpura, cutaneous infections, telogen effluvium, hirsutism, acanthosis nigricans

Table 2. Side Effects of corticosteroids[10]

The primary consideration in treating vitiligo is careful patient selection in order to maximize response to vitiligo while minimizing adverse effects. The other concern is determination of proper dose and dosing schedule.

Side effects can be dose- or duration-dependent. Dose-dependent side effects of corticosteroids are hyperglycemia, hyperlipidemia, peptic ulcer disease, and psychosis. Duration-dependent changes are hypertension, cushingoid changes, growth impairment, osteoporosis, osteonecrosis and opportunistic infections.[10] Steroid withdrawal syndrome is observed when systemic corticosteroids given at high doses are abruptly stopped and it presents as vague symptoms of lethargy, generalized weakness and myalgia. Abrupt withdrawal of the corticosteroid does not give enough time for the suppressed HPA axis to recover. It is observed with doses higher than 20-30 mg of prednisolone. Duration of treatment is not a predictable causative factor.[28] High dose of corticosteroid can also lead to extreme suppression of adrenals (Addisonian crisis) manifesting as hypotension and extreme weakness. Cushingoid changes occur with long term treatment and present as puffiness of face, moon facies, buffalo hump, striae, increased hair growth on face, skin atrophy, increased abdominal girth with thin extremities and others. Growth impairment and opportunistic infections can be decreased by avoiding daily administration either by using alternate day dosing or OMP. Oral mini pulse therapy has fewer side effects (*e.g.*, moon facies, weight gain, acne) compared to daily dosing as reviewed in a meta-analysis.[29] Betamethasone and dexamethasone can be used interchangeably as the potency and half-life are almost same. When compared to other corticosteroids, deflazacort is considered to have relatively fewer cases of growth retardation in children, osteoporosis, weight gain and HPA axis suppression.[11]

Absolute contraindications to use of systemic corticosteroids are very few, and include such conditions as systemic fungal infections and herpes simplex keratitis. Relative contraindications are congestive heart failure, human immunodeficiency virus (HIV), psychosis, active peptic ulcer disease, active tuberculosis, and septicemia. Well-controlled diabetes and hypertension are not contraindications, but lower doses should be used, the concomitant disease must be adequately treated, and the patient should be monitored frequently.

There are various approaches to minimize the side effects of corticosteroids. First is to give corticosteroids only as long as disease activity is present and the taper it slowly (over a period of 3-6 months) when no indication of new lesions are present. The oral mini pulse therapy regimen has significantly less side effects compared to typical daily dosing of corticosteroids. An important finding is the lack of prolonged HPA axis suppression with OMP therapy.[22] Furthermore, higher doses of dexamethasone (10 mg) do not seem to provide any additional benefit to 5 mg betamethasone.[9, 22] Choosing corticosteroids with less risk of mineralocorticoid-type effects (*i.e.*, dexamethasone, betamethasone) or one with supposedly fewer side effects (*i.e.*, deflazacort) can be beneficial for all patients. Calcium supplementation, salt restriction, proper diet, daily exercise and use of antacids can minimize risk of side effects. Regular monitoring of weight, fasting blood sugar, and blood pressure will help in early detection of side effects if they occur.

8. Safety in children and pregnancy

The decision to treat progressive vitiligo in children below 4 years of age can be rather difficult as limited data is available for this population. It is suggested that oral mini pulse therapy be modified (*i.e.*, 1 mg of dexamethasone or betamethasone given for every 10 kg) and used.

Corticosteroids have been safely used in pregnancy and are classified as category C drugs (animal reproduction studies have shown an adverse effect on the fetus and there are no adequate and well-controlled studies in humans, but potential benefits may warrant use of the drug in pregnant women despite potential risks). However, it is best to reserve its use in pregnancy when the benefits of treatment outweigh the risk of side effects. Pregnancy is known to precipitate and aggravate vitiligo. However, vitiligo being a non-life threatening condition, a patient may defer any type of treatment, including corticosteroids.

9. Efficacy of corticosteroids in vitiligo

Worldwide, there are few studies published documenting the efficacy and safety of corticosteroids in vitiligo. The available reports are primarily case series and there is a lack of well validated randomized controlled trials.

9.1 Oral mini pulse therapy

Pasricha *et al* evaluated the effect of five different regimens in causing repigmentation and stopping disease activity for four months and noted that regimens using corticosteroids were superior to those excluding corticosteroids. Improvement with 3 mg betamethasone orally on alternate days combined with levamisole and topical fluocinolone, 2 mg betamethasone orally alternating with 20 mg 8-methoxypsoralen and sun exposure, and oral mini pulse consisting of 5 mg betamethasone orally twice a week combined with 50 mg cyclophosphamide daily orally was 87.5%, 85% and 90.9% respectively, while levamisole 150 mg two days a week showed improvement in 53.8%. Addition of topical fluocinolone acetonide to levamisole showed better response in 81.8%.[8]

In a study on forty patients by Pasricha and Khaitan, 5 mg betamethasone as a single oral dose after breakfast on 2 consecutive days per week was found effective in halting disease progression in 89% patients within 1-3 months and inducing variable spontaneous repigmentation in patients with extensive and rapidly progressive disease.[9] Only 2 patients did not show response initially, but once the dose was increased from 5 mg to 7.5 mg, there was notable improvement. Side effects were seen in 23%(17) patients, such as weight gain (5), mild headache (2), transient general weakness (2), bad taste in mouth (3), acne (2) and mild puffiness, perioral dermatitis, as well as herpes zoster, glaucoma and amenorrhea, of which were reported in one patient each. Kanwar *et al*[23]and Radakovic-Fijan *et al*[22] also reported efficacy of dexamethasone oral mini pulse therapy in arresting progression of rapidly spreading vitiligo in 43.8% and 88%, respectively. The difference in response in this study by Kanwar *et al* and the one conducted by Pasricha and Khaitan could be because of the higher proportion of patients with segmental vitiligo and shorter duration of treatment in the Kanwar *et al* study.

OMP has been found to be effective in patients with unstable generalized and acrofacial vitiligo in a randomized double-blind placebo-controlled randomized prospective study.[30]

Prednisolone has been used as once a week oral dose of 2 mg/kg in 50 patients with extensive and rapidly spreading vitiligo. The disease progression was arrested in 93% and repigmentation observed in 88% with only 3 patients developing side effects.[31] Methylprednisolone 0.8mg/kg given as OMP along with topical fluticasone in children for 6 months was safe and effective in arresting disease in 90% and producing variable repigmentation in 65%.[32]

OMP in combination with other standard vitiligo treatments has also been studied. Betamethasone has been used as an adjunct to surgery for treatment of stable vitiligo patches in patients who did not respond to their first surgical.[24] It has also been combined with phototherapy and photochemotherapy. Dexamethasone OMP has been found effective and safe with psoralen with solar ultraviolet light (PUVAsol) in fast spreading vitiligo.[30] OMP has been safely used in children and was more effective than 8-methoxypsoralen alone.[33] Combination of narrowband UVB (NB-UVB) with OMP has been compared with psoralen and ultraviolet A (PUVA) photochemotherapy with OMP. Disease progression is arrested in both, but repigmentation was better and earlier with NB-UVB.[34]

Immunosuppressants can also be added to OMP. A comparison study of three regimens: (a) OMP with daily cyclophosphamide, (b) a 3-day dexamethasone-cyclophosphamide pulse given monthly, and (c) daily cyclophosphamide and dexamethasone-cyclophosphamide pulse given only on one day in a month showed that disease activity was arrested by all three modalities but repigmentation up to 75% was seen in 71%, 62%, and 53%, respectively. The higher response with OMP may be because weekly dosing may provide better immunosuppression in the context of vitiligo as compared to monthly dosing in pulse therapy.[35] Weight gain was more frequent with OMP, but otherwise all three regimens had a similar frequency of side effects.[35]

9.2 Daily corticosteroids

In everyday practice, corticosteroids are primarily administered daily at doses individualized for each specific patient. Published studies are based on prednisolone given at 0.3mg/kg as a single oral dose after breakfast initially for the first 2 months. The dosage is then reduced to half the initial dose during at the third month and halved again in at the fourth month of treatment. With this regimen, Kim *et al* noted that disease progression was halted in 87.7% of patients and in 70.4%, repigmentation was also seen.[26] In a study by Banerjee *et al*, disease progression was arrested in 90% and repigmentation was seen in 76%.[27] The side effects observed in both studies were not serious, and did not warrant a change in dose or dosing schedule. Disease was also reported to completely subside after discontinuing treatment in addition to other positive observations; this suggests that low dose corticosteroids given for 4 months may be reasonably safe and effective treatment option.

9.3 Intravenous pulse therapy

Methylprednisolone (8 mg/kg) given intravenously on three consecutive days a month was used in a study as pulse therapy in 14 patients with generalized vitiligo. Eighty-five percent of the patients who presented with progressive disease showed cessation of disease progression and 71% of these patients had repigmentation. None of the six patients presenting with static disease showed any repigmentation. The therapy was well tolerated in all but one patient who developed intermittent arterial hypertension during therapy.[36]

Most studies indicate that systemic corticosteroids are helpful in halting disease progression in rapidly spreading vitiligo and inducing spontaneous repigmentation. However their role in static vitiligo is not well documented. As of now, corticosteroids can be recommended for rapidly spreading vitiligo for a short duration to halt disease activity, but it should not be used for repigmentation in static vitiligo, even if disease is extensive. Areas that require further research is the risk of osteoporosis with corticosteroids and the efficacy of calcium supplementation. Studies with longer follow-up periods are required to evaluate the potential for relapse. Deflazacort needs to be evaluated as a relatively safer corticosteroid option for vitiligo since its use in vitiligo is very limited. Head-to-head comparative studies between betamethasone, prednisolone, and deflazacort may be useful for determining the optimal agent for treatment.

10. Conclusion

There seems to be a definite role for systemic corticosteroids in the treatment of vitiligo. The types of vitiligo in which benefits have been observed are: (a) rapidly progressing vitiligo, (b) slowly progressing vitiligo with extensive involvement and frequent exacerbation, (c) frank inflammatory vitiligo, (d) patients with direct or indirect evidence of autoimmune disease (*e.g.,* high titers of thyroid autoantibodies), (d) recalcitrant static vitiligo with exacerbation, and (e) rescue therapy. Corticosteroids should not usually be considered for universal vitiligo, segmental vitiligo or focal limited vitiligo.

Although daily or alternate day oral corticosteroids may be treatment options, OMP therapy seems to be the best regimen for long-term use with minimal side effects. The duration of OMP should be at least 6 months or longer and tapering to discontinuation should be slow and step-wise. When a patient is on any regimen that includes systemic corticosteroids, regular and periodic monitoring must be done to assess the risk-to-benefit ratio of treatment and to evaluate efficacy. Further study is needed to provide more definitive evidence for systemic corticosteroid use in vitiligo as well as the long-term implications of treatment.

11. References

[1] Majumdar PP. Genetics and prevalence of vitiligo vulgaris. In: Hann SK, Nordlund JJ, Editors. Vitiligo. 2000, Blackwell Science Ltd. p. 18-20.

[2] Mattoo SK, Handa S, Kaur I, Gupta N, Malhotra R. Psychiatric morbidity in vitiligo: prevalence and correlates in India. J Eur Acad Dermatol Venereol 2002; 16: 573-8.
[3] Linthorst Homan MW, Spuls PI, de Korte J, Bos JD, Sprangers MA, van der Veen JP. The burden of vitiligo: patient characteristics associated with quality of life. J Am Acad Dermatol. 2009; 61: 411-20.
[4] Pasricha JS, Khaitan BK. Drugs for vitiligo. New Age International (P) limited, 1996, New Delhi. p. 37-43.
[5] Farah FS, Kurban AK, Chaglassian HT. The treatment of vitiligo with psoralens and triamcinolone by mouth. Br J Dermatol 1967; 79: 89-91.
[6] Gokhale BB, Gokhale TB. Corticotrophin and vitiligo (preliminary observations). Br J Dermatol. 1976; 95: 329.
[7] Imamura S, Tagami H. Treatment of vitiligo with oral corticosteroids. Dermatologica. 1976; 153: 179-85.
[8] Pasricha JS, Seetharam KA, Dashore A. Evaluation of five different regimes for the treatment of vitiligo. Indian J Dermatol Venereol 1989; 55: 18-21.
[9] Pasricha JS, Khaitan BK. Oral mini-pulse therapy with betamethasone in vitiligo patients having extensive or fast-spreading disease.Int J Dermatol. 1993; 32: 753-7.
[10] Wolverton SE. Systemic corticosteroids. In :Wolverton SE. Comprehensive dermatologic drug therapy. 2nd edition. Saunders Elseviers, Philadelphia. 2007. p 127-61.
[11] Joshi N, Rajeshwari K. Deflazacort. J Postgrad Med 2009; 55: 296-300.
[12] Abdel-Naser MB, Krüger-Krasagakes S, Krasagakis K, Gollnick H, Abdel-Fattah A, Orfanos CE. Further evidence for involvement of both cell mediated and humoral immunity in generalized vitiligo. Pigment Cell Res. 1994; 7: 1-8.
[13] Ahn SK, Choi EH, Lee SH, Won JH, Hann SK, Park YK. Immunohistochemical studies from vitiligo--comparison between active and inactive lesions. Yonsei Med J. 1994; 35: 404-10.
[14] Abdel-Naser MB, Ludwig WD, Gollnick H, Orfanos CE. Nonsegmental vitiligo: decrease of the CD45RA+ T-cell subset and evidence for peripheral T-cell activation. Int J Dermatol. 1992; 31: 321-6.
[15] Ogg GS, Rod Dunbar P, Romero P, Chen JL, Cerundolo V. High frequency of skin-homing melanocyte-specific cytotoxic T lymphocytes in autoimmune vitiligo. J Exp Med. 1998; 188: 1203-8.
[16] Wańkowicz-Kalińska A, van den Wijngaard RM, Tigges BJ, Westerhof W, Ogg GS,etal. Immunopolarization of CD4+ and CD8+ T cells to Type-1-like is associated with melanocyte loss in human vitiligo. Lab Invest. 2003; 83: 683-95.
[17] van den Boorn JG, Konijnenberg D, Dellemijn TA, van der Veen JP, Bos JD, Melief CJ, Vyth-Dreese FA, Luiten RM. Autoimmune destruction of skin melanocytes by perilesional T cells from vitiligo patients. J Invest Dermatol. 2009; 129: 2220-32.
[18] Klarquist J, Denman CJ, Hernandez C, Wainwright DA, Strickland FM, Overbeck A, etal. Reduced skin homing by functional Treg in vitiligo. Pigment Cell Melanoma Res. 2010; 23: 276-86.
[19] Hann SK, Kim HI, Im S, Park YK, Cui J, Bystryn JC. The change of melanocyte cytotoxicity after systemic steroid treatment in vitiligo patients J Dermatol Sci. 1993; 6: 201-5.
[20] Lee DY, Choi SC, Lee JH. Generalized vitiligo treated by combination therapy of epidermal graft and systemic corticosteroid. Clin Exp Dermatol. 2009; 34: 838.

[21] Lee DY, Lee KJ, Choi SC, Lee JH. Segmental vitiligo treated by the combination of epidermal grafting and systemic corticosteroids. Dermatol Surg. 2010; 36: 575-6.

[22] Radakovic-Fijan S, Fürnsinn-Friedl AM, Hönigsmann H, TanewA. Oral dexamethasone pulse treatment for vitiligo. J Am Acad Dermatol. 2001; 44: 814-7.

[23] Kanwar AJ, Dhar S, Dawn G. Oral minipulse therapy in vitiligo.Dermatology1995; 190: 251-2.

[24] Mulekar SV. Stable vitiligo treated by a combination of low-dose oral pulse betamethasone and autologous, noncultured melanocyte-keratinocyte cell transplantation. Dermatol Surg. 2006; 32: 536-41.

[25] Seiter S, Ugurel S, Pföhler C, Tilgen W, Reinhold U. Successful treatment of progressive vitiligo with high-dose intravenous methylprednisolone 'pulse' therapy. Dermatology. 1999; 199: 261-2.

[26] Kim SM, Lee HS, Hann SK. The efficacy of low-dose oral corticosteroids in the treatment of vitiligo patients. Int J Dermatol 1999; 38: 546-50.

[27] Banerjee K, Barbhuiya JN, Ghosh AP, Dey SK, Karmakar PR. The efficacy of low-dose oral corticosteroids in the treatment of vitiligo patient. Indian J Dermatol Venereol Leprol. 2003; 69: 135-7.

[28] Daly JR, Myles AB, Bacon PA, Beardwell CG, Savage O. pituitary adrenal function during corticosteroid withdrwal in rheumatoid arthritis. Ann Theum Dis 1967; 26; 18-25.

[29] Njoo MD, Spuls PI, Bos JD, Westerhof W, Bossuyt PM. Non-surgical repigmentation therapies in vitiligo. Meta-analysis of the literature. Arch Dermatol. 1998; 134: 1532-40.

[30] Paul M *et al*. OMP steroid therapy in the treatment of unstable vitiligo-a double blind placebo controlled randomized prospective study. Presented at 26th Annual Conference of IADVL, 1998.

[31] Gupta RR. Modified oral mini pulse steroid therapy in unstable vitiligo-A novel once a week regimen. Presented at 29th Annual Conference of IADVL, 2001.

[32] Imran M *et al*. Childhood vitiligo: Response to methylprednisolone OMP therapy and topical fluticasone preparation. Indian J Dermatol 2010; 54: 124-7.

[33] Nigam PK. Clinical and oral minipulse therapy evaluation in childhood vitiligo. Presented at 32th Annual Conference of IADVL, 2004.

[34] Rath N *et al*. PUVA vs NB(UVB) with OMP: efficacy in progressive vitiligo. Presented at 32nd Annual Conference IADVL, 2004.

[35] Singh YL, Khaitan BK, Ramam M, Pasricha JS. A comparative study of the effect of three regimens comprising of corticosteroids and cyclophosphamide for the treatment of vitiligo. Thesis submitted to AIIMS, June 1999 (unpublished).

[36] Seiter S, Ugurel S, Tilgen W, Reinhold U. Use of high-dose methylprednisolone pulse therapy in patients with progressive and stable vitiligo. Int J Dermatol. 2000; 39: 624-7.

7

Segmental Vitiligo

Ji-Hye Park and Dong-Youn Lee
Department of Dermatology, Samsung Medical Center
Sungkyunkwan University, Seoul
South Korea

1. Introduction

Vitiligo is largely classified into segmental and non-segmental types (Table 1).[1] This classification is based on the original report by Koga in 1977.[2] Koga proposed that vitiligo in a non-dermatomal distribution be referred to as *Type A* and vitiligo in a dermatomal distribution be *Type B*, the latter of which corresponds to what is known today as **segmental vitiligo (SV)**. Since then, the distinctive characteristics of SV have been described.[3-6] Recently, it was proposed that vitiligo be classified into four major types: segmental, non-segmental, mixed, and unclassified.[7]

The incidence of SV is not well-established because different investigators report variable percentages of patients having SV. El-Mofty *et al* reported that only 5% of patients with vitiligo had the segmental type.[8] Koga and Tango described that in their population, 27.9% had SV.3 Several studies in Korea revealed the prevalence of SV to range from 5.5% to 29.6%.[4,9,10]

The typical lesion of SV is not significantly different from that of NSV. Both can initially appear as focal vitiligo, which involves a small area.[11] However, SV has a distinct natural history and unique clinical features.[1,3,4] In addition, SV shows different therapeutic characteristics when compared with NSV.[1,12]

SV can appear at any age, but the majority of cases occur early in life between the ages of 5 and 30 years old. Koga and Tango reported that 82% of type B vitiligo (SV) patients noticed their first depigmented patches before the age of 30.[3] In the pivotal SV study by Hann and Lee, the mean age of onset was 15.6 years, and SV developed before 10 years of age in 41% of cases, and before 30 years of age in 87%.[4] In our study, the mean age of onset was 19.8 years; 32% of SV started before 10 years of age and 62% before 20 years of age.[6]

SV typically presents with unilateral involvement of depigmented macules surrounded by normal skin. The color of the macules is usually white and more distinguishable with Wood's light examination. However, macules may have a more irregular border and less homogeneous pattern of pigment loss than NSV.[11] Trichrome vitiligo, which is characterized by both depigmented and hypopigmented macules, is reported in SV.[13]

SV shows a quasi-dermatomal mode of distribution, but seems to be different from the pattern of herpes zoster. SV often involves a segment that includes the parts of several dermatomes and may at times, go over the midline partially. Some cases may involve lines or large bands consistent with Blaschko's lines.[14,15] There is no preferential distribution between right and left sides of the body. Very rarely, SV involves two or more different segments with ipsilateral or contralateral distribution. Lee and Hann reported that 5 of 240 SV cases showed bilateral SV on the same or different dermatomes that appeared on both sides of the body.[16]

The face is the most common site of SV regardless of gender (Figure 1). According to the Hann and Lee study, 51% of SV involved the face, 25% the trunk (Figure 2), and 11% the extremities. In our own study, 54% of SV involved only the face.[4] An additional 17% had both face and neck involvement of SV (Figure 3).[6]

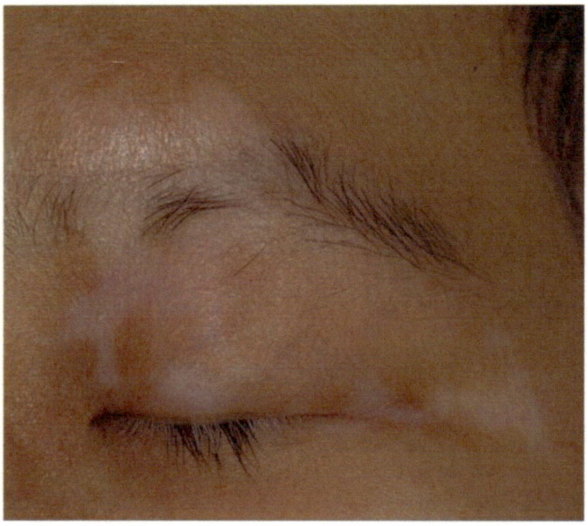

Fig. 1. Segmental vitiligo on the face.

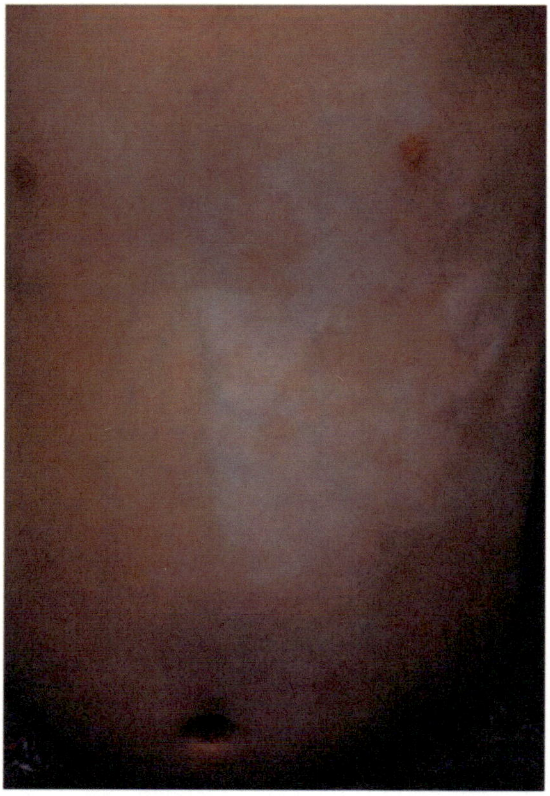

Fig. 2. Segmental vitiligo on the abdomen.

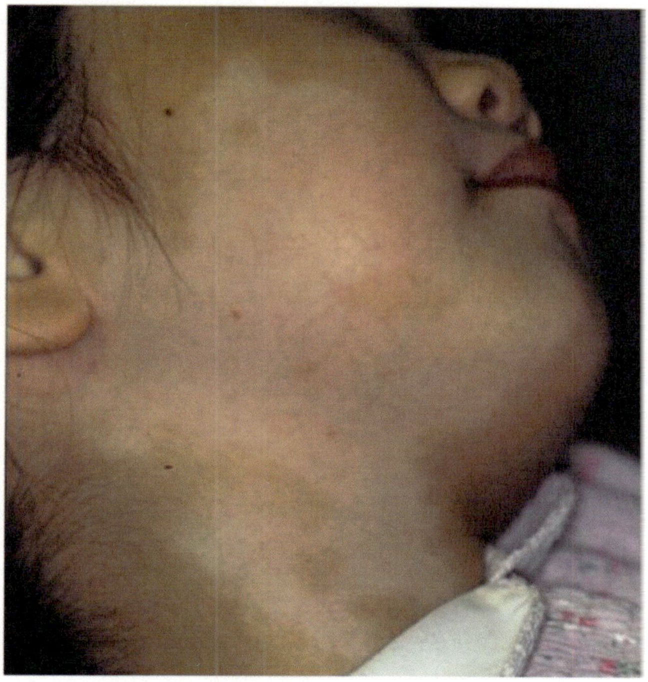

Fig. 3. Segmental vitiligo on the face and neck.

Hann *et al* proposed the original classification of the SV distribution of the face.[17] This was revised to include 6 types depending on pattern and area of involvement.[15] This classification may be valuable for certain aspects of prognosis, such as the likely degree and path of lesional spread.

SV is often associated with the occurrence of white hair (*i.e.,* poliosis, leukotrichia) in lesional skin. SV tends to involve the hair compartment soon after onset compared to NSV.[1] Hann and Lee reported that poliosis was found in 49% of 208 patients with SV.[4] The eyebrow (Figure 4) and eyelashes commonly show white hair and other hair-bearing sites including the scalp, pubis, and axilla can be involved. However, it is very difficult to notice the presence of white hairs on other areas of the body with the naked eye because the hairs consist of tiny, thin vellus hairs. We examined 82 patients for the presence of leukotrichia in SV lesions using a digital portable microscope. All of the patients demonstrated leukotrichia independent of age and disease duration (Figure 5).[6,18] The amount of white hair was variable. These results suggest that a very high percentage of patients with SV have associated leukotrichia.

It has been reported that SV usually spreads within a segment in a short period of time and then tends to stop.[3,4] However, in our own study, we observed 87 patients who had SV for mean of 29.5 months (maximum 150 months), 19 cases (21.8%) showed disease progression 4 years after disease onset (2011 IPCC presentation). Therefore, more long-term follow-up data are needed in order to more accurately understand the natural course and the long-term recurrence rate of SV.

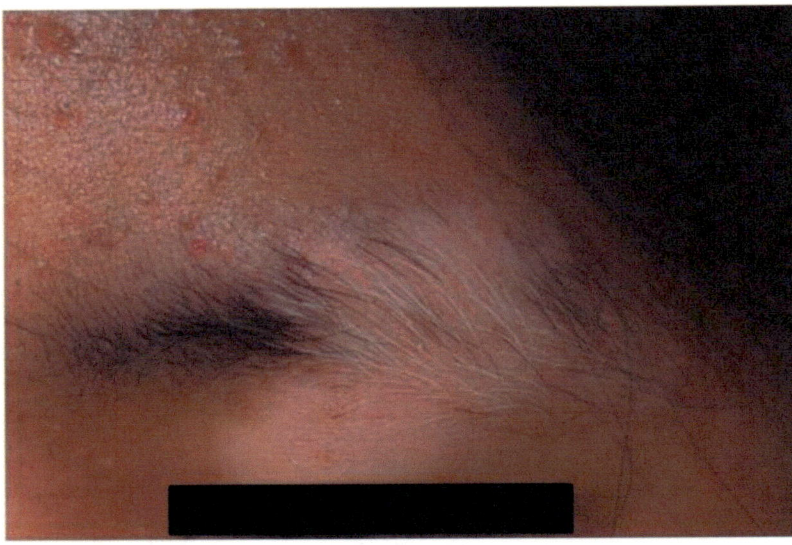

Fig. 4. White hairs of the eyebrow in segmental vitiligo can be seen.

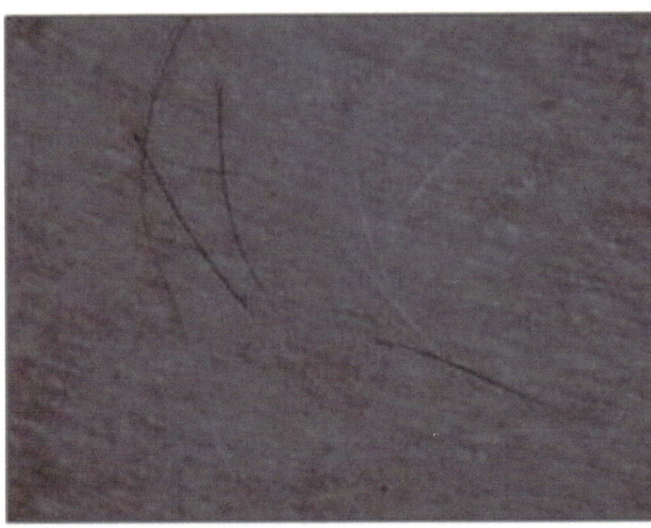

Fig. 5. Leukotrichia in a segmental vitiligo lesion can be seen easily using portable digital microscopy (magnified 30x)

It has been proposed that the rare instance of SV progresses into a generalized form, that this be called mixed vitiligo.[19] However, this likely represents only the rare circumstance of concurrent SV and NSV rather than its own independent vitiligo type.

SV is not usually accompanied by other autoimmune diseases contrary to NSV.[1,3,8] However, Park *et al* reported that about 9.5% of SV cases were associated with other diseases[20] and Hann *et al* described that 6.7% of 208 patients had an associated disease, including atopic dermatitis, halo nevus, thyroid disease, diabetes mellitus, and alopecia areata.[4]

Segmental Vitiligo	Non-Segmental Vitiligo
Often early age of onset	Variable age of onset
Usually unilateral	Usually bilateral
Is known to spread rapidly and stabilize in a few years*	Usually chronic and progressive course
Predictable course	Unpredictable course
Very high percentage of white hairs (leukotrichia) of lesional skin in early stage disease	Variable percentage of white hairs (leukotrichia) of lesional skin
Shows good response to autologous grafting	Shows unpredictable results after autologous grafting
Is not usually associated with autoimmune disease	Is often associated with personal or family history of autoimmune disease

*Long-term data is still warranted.

Table 1. Comparison of Segmental Vitiligo and Non-Segmental Vitiligo

2. Treatment of segmental vitiligo

Segmental vitiligo (SV) is a distinct type of vitiligo in terms of its clinical features, natural course, and response to treatment, that make it distinguishable from non-segmental vitiligo (NSV).[1,2] In SV, white macules are usually localized to one segment on only one side of the body, however, in NSV white macules can occur at any body location and disease activity tends to persist throughout the life of the patient. Thus, the course of SV is predictable while that of NSV is unpredictable. Treatment guidelines of SV may be easier to determine than those of NSV.

Until now, many articles about vitiligo treatment have been published. However, many of these studies were not randomized, controlled, and double-blinded, but rather retrospective studies or case reports. In addition, many studies did not distinguish between the types of vitiligo or they did not provide demographic information about SV in detail. Thus, reliable publications about the treatment of SV are scarce.

The treatment modalities for vitiligo largely consist of medical and surgical therapies.[21] Medical management includes topical corticosteroids and immunomodulators, and phototherapy such as narrow-band UVB (NB-UVB) and excimer laser. If medical treatment is unsatisfactory, surgical treatments such as autologous skin grafting may be considered. Taïeb and Picardo presented treatment guidelines for vitiligo in a review.[1]

2.1 Topical corticosteroids

Topical corticosteroids have been used for the treatment of vitiligo for decades. There have only been a few studies about the effects of topical corticosteroids in SV.

Koga evaluated the effect of topical corticosteroids in vitiligo patients.[2] In this study, only five patients with SV were included and received topical steroid therapy (0.12% betamethasone-17-valerate, 0.01% fluocinolone acetonide, or 0.1% triamcinolone acetonide cream or ointment) for a minimum of 2 months. However, no improvement was found in any of these patients.

Khalid and Mujtaba treated forty SV patients with 0.05% clobetasol propionate cream twice daily.[22] Therapy was interrupted every 6 weeks for a 2-week treatment-free period. Some response was observed in the majority of patients (79%, 30 out of 38) and more than 50% repigmentation was observed in 34% (13) of patients. The best results were found on the face. Out of the 23 patients who presented within 1 year of SV onset, 11 (47.8%) showed more than 50% repigmentation; on the other hand, only two out of 15 (13.3%) patients who presented after one year of the onset of SV achieved the same degree of response. The side effects were mild skin atrophy in six patients, telangiectasias in four patients, and acneiform papules in eight patients. These results suggest that disease duration may be an important indicator of prognosis because most of the patients showing more than 50% repigmentation presented within one year of SV onset.

2.2 Topical immunomodulators (calcineurin inhibitors)

Several studies have demonstrated the efficacy of tacrolimus ointment and pimecrolimus cream in the treatment of vitiligo patients. However, most of them did not disclose the inclusion of SV.

Silverberg *et al* assessed the efficacy of topical tacrolimus ointment in the treatment of childhood vitiligo.[23] Fifty-seven patients were treated with tacrolimus ointment (0.03% or 0.1%) once or twice daily for a minimum of three months. In their series, 37% of the patients had SV, most commonly of the head and/or neck. Among the SV patients, 86% responded to tacrolimus ointment, especially those with facial involvement (94%). One patient showed complete repigmentation on the chin and neck after eight weeks of summer sun exposure along with twice daily tacrolimus 0.03% ointment.

Udompataikul *et al* evaluated the effectiveness of 0.1% tacrolimus ointment in 42 vitiligo patients, of whom eleven patients had SV.[24] The overall response rate, defined as at least some evidence of repigmentation, was 76% and the response rate for SV was 77%.

2.3 Phototherapy

Phototherapy has been widely used for the treatment of vitiligo. However, most studies about phototherapy in vitiligo were performed in patients with NSV.

1. NB-UVB

Anbar *et al* evaluated the clinical response of vitiligo patients to NB-UVB. Their study included 150 patients with SV (10%) or NSV (90%).[25] NB-UVB therapy was given twice weekly. In the NSV group, 48% of patients showed a marked response (more than 75% repigmentation) and 27% showed a moderate response (between 26% and 75% repigmentation). However, in the SV group, 92.3 % showed no more than a mild response (less than 25% repigmentation) to treatment regardless of the lesion site, and only 7.7% of SV patients showed a moderate response.

NB-UVB microphototherapy uses a device that delivers a focused beam with wavelengths from 300 to 320 nanometers (nm) with a peak emission of 311 nm. Lotti *et al* evaluated the effectiveness of UVB microphototherapy for eight SV patients for six months.[26] Five patients achieved normal pigmentation on more than 75% of their treated areas.

2. PUVA

Tallab *et al* evaluated the efficacy of systemic psoralen and ultraviolet A (PUVA) in the treatment of vitiligo retrospectively.[27] Thirty-two patients with vitiligo were studied, including five patients with SV. All of the SV patients showed no or poor repigmentation. They concluded that SV was very resistant to PUVA therapy.

3. Excimer laser

The 308 nm excimer laser has demonstrated promising efficacy and appealing side effect profile for localized vitiligo.[28,29] Compared with conventional NB-UVB, excimer laser generally provides more rapid repigmentation in limited forms of vitiligo.

Do *et al* performed a retrospective analysis to evaluate the treatment response to excimer laser in SV patients.[30] Eighty patients with SV were included. Repigmentation was graded as: grade 0, no repigmentation; grade 1, 1–24%; grade 2, 25–49%; grade 3, 50–74%; grade 4, 75–99%; grade 5, complete repigmentation. The mean grade of repigmentation was 2.3 after a mean of 20.6 months of treatment; 23.8% showed grade 4, 20% showed grade 3, and 56.2% showed grade 1–2 repigmentation. However, none of them achieved complete repigmentation. They observed that SV had a better repigmentation response rate when the excimer laser was used at earlier stages of the disease for longer treatment durations with high cumulative UV energy. However, the limitation of their study was that many patients received other concurrent treatments such as oral corticosteroids, topical steroids, or topical tacrolimus ointment during the study period.

4. Miscellaneous Therapies

We retrospectively evaluated the effect of phototherapy in nine patients with SV depending on the disease duration.[31] All patients except one had SV for longer than two years when they started on a phototherapy regimen of PUVA, NB-UVB, or excimer laser. All patients showed a poor response to phototherapy irrespective of the type of phototherapy administered. Our results suggest that phototherapy is not helpful in long-duration SV.

It has been reported that the combination of NB-UVB and tacrolimus ointment is effective in vitiligo.[32] However, this combination treatment of NB-UVB and tacrolimus ointment in SV is limited to case reports.

We presented two cases of recent onset SV that showed good or excellent response to targeted phototherapy (Dualight®) in combination with drug therapy.[33] Our results suggest that SV can be improved with combination therapy if SV onset is recent, emphasizing that early treatment may be essential for this type of vitiligo. In addition, we reported a case of SV that showed a marked response to combination NB-UVB and 0.1% topical tacrolimus compared with 0.1% topical tacrolimus alone.[34] This case suggests that combination therapy is necessary for SV.

Low-energy helium-neon laser (632.8 nm) has applications in a variety of clinical conditions including vitiligo. Yu *et al* evaluated the efficacy of the helium-neon laser on thirty patients with SV on the head and/or neck.[35] Marked repigmentation (more than 50%) was observed in 60% of patients.

2.4 Surgical treatment

Generally, surgical treatment is indicated for stable vitiligo that does not respond to medical treatment.[36] Patients with SV are considered a good candidates for surgical treatment.[21] Although medical treatment is often helpful in SV, complete repigmentation is almost always difficult to obtain. Thus, surgical treatment is necessary for complete repigmentation in many cases of SV. Surgical treatment includes autologous epidermal grafting (Figure 6), mini-grafting, and transplantation of epidermal cell suspensions.[21]

Gupta and Kumar analyzed a retrospective, uncontrolled case series and literature review of 143 patients treated with epidermal grafting. They found that repigmentation success rates for generalized and segmental (including focal) vitiligo were 53 and 91%, respectively.[37]

In epidermal grafting surgeries, oral corticosteroids may be a helpful adjunct. We reported that in a case of SV with failure to repigment with surgery alone, that response occurred when oral corticosteroid was added to the grafting procedure.[38] In addition, we also presented that achieving better results in SV may be contingent on combination therapy utilizing epidermal grafting with systemic corticosteroids.[39]

SV may continue to spread even a few years after onset of disease. We presented a case of SV which continued to spread after epidermal grafting; the new lesions did not involve the area of previous epidermal grafting, but repeated epidermal grafting was successful.[40] This case indicates that epidermal grafting can be useful for the treatment of SV although recurrence may arise.

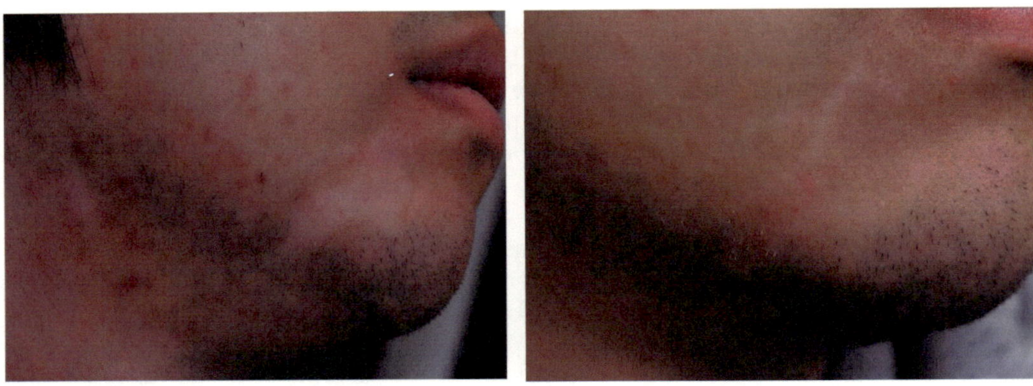

Fig. 6. Before (left) and after (right) epidermal grafting in segmental vitiligo.

In vitiligo lesions with leukotrichia present, the possibility of repigmentation may be minimal or absent because the loss of hair melanocytes is usually permanent, and repigmentation may not occur even with medical treatment. We found that the majority of white hairs in SV may contribute to the lack of response to medical treatment and require surgical treatment such as epidermal grafting.[6]

First-Line
- Topical treatment (topical corticosteroids, calcineurin inhibitors) and narrow-band UVB (NB-UVB) therapy or targeted phototherapy (*i.e.*, excimer laser) for at least 3 months. If there is treatment response, continue the regimen for 1 year.
- If the majority of hairs in the lesional skin are white (leukotrichia), consider surgical treatment.
Second-Line
- Consider surgical treatment if medical treatment is unsatisfactory.

Table 2. Treatment Guidelines for Segmental Vitiligo

Based on previous reports and our experiences, we recently proposed a set of treatment guidelines in SV.[12] Treatments such as topical corticosteroids and topical calcineurin inhibitors, as well as phototherapy, including NB-UVB and targeted phototherapy (*e.g.*, excimer laser) are helpful for SV.[23,26,30] Available data suggests that combination topical treatment and phototherapy is more efficacious in SV than any type of monotherapy.[33,34] In addition, disease duration in SV is very important to consider to gauge response to medical treatment.[22,24,30] Thus, as first-line therapy, we recommend the combination of topical treatment and phototherapy to be initiated as early as possible. However, our experience suggests that phototherapy is not helpful in SV patients with the majority of hairs in lesional skin being white.[6] Therefore, in these cases, we recommend first-line treatment be surgery in order to avoid delay as well as unnecessary and inefficacious treatment. These guidelines will contribute to future definitive treatment guidelines for SV (Table 2).

3. References

[1] Taïeb A, Picardo M. Clinical practice. Vitiligo. N Engl J Med 2009;360:160-169

[2] Koga M. Vitiligo: a new classification and therapy. Br J Dermatol 1977;97:255-261

[3] Koga M, Tango T. Clinical features and course of type A and type B vitiligo. Br J Dermatol 1988;118:223-228

[4] Hann SK, Lee HJ. Segmental vitiligo: clinical findings in 208 patients. J Am Acad Dermatol 1996;35:671-674

[5] Mazereeuw-Hautier J, Bezio S, Mahe E, et al. Segmental and nonsegmental childhood vitiligo has distinct clinical characteristics: a prospective observational study. J Am Acad Dermatol. 2010;62:945-9.

[6] Lee DY, Kim CR, Park JH, et al. The incidence of leukotrichia in segmental vitiligo: implication of poor response to medical treatment. Int J Dermatol 2011;50:925-927

[7] Taïeb A, Picardo M. Epidemiology, definitions and classification. In: Picardo M, Taïeb A, eds. Vitiligo, 1st edn. Berlin: Springer, 2010: 13–24.

[8] El-Mofty AM, el-Mofty M. Vitiligo. A symptom complex. Int J Dermatol 1980;19:237-244

[9] Song MS HS, Ahn PS, Im S, Park YK. Clinical study of vitiligo: Comparative study of type A and type B vitiligo. Ann Dermatol 1994;6:22-30

[10] Bang JS Lee JW, Kim TH, et al. Comparative clinical study of segmental and non-segmental vitiligo. Kor J Dermatol 2000;38:1037-1044

[11] Taïeb A, Picardo M. The definition and assessment of vitiligo: a consensus report of the Vitiligo European Task Force. Pigment Cell Res 2007;20:27-35

[12] Lee DY, Choi SC. A proposal for the treatment guideline in segmental vitiligo. Int J Dermatol 2011 in press

[13] Lee DY, Kim CR, Lee JH. Trichrome vitiligo in segmental type. Photodermatol Photoimmunol Photomed 2011;27:111-112

[14] Taïeb A, Morice-Picard F, Jouary T, et al. Segmental vitiligo as the possible expression of cutaneous somatic mosaicism: implications for common non-segmental vitiligo. Pigment Cell Melanoma Res 2008;21:646-652

[15] Kim DY, Oh SH, Hann SK. Classification of segmental vitiligo on the face: clues for prognosis. Br J Dermatol 2011;164:1004-1009

[16] Lee HS, Hann SK. Bilateral segmental vitiligo. Ann Dermatol 1998;10:129-131

[17] Hann SK, Chang JH, Lee HS, et al. The classification of segmental vitiligo on the face. Yonsei Med J 2000;41:209-212

[18] Lee DY, Park JH, Lee JH, et al. Is segmental vitiligo always associated with leukotrichia? Examination with a digital portable microscope. Int J Dermatol 2009;48:1262.

[19] Ezzedine K, Gauthier Y, Leaute-Labreze C, et al. Segmental vitiligo associated with generalized vitiligo (mixed vitiligo): A retrospective case series of 19 patients. J Am Acad Dermatol 2011 in pres

[20] Park KC, Youn JI, Lee YS. Clinical study of 326 cases of vitiligo. Korean J Dermatol 1988;26:200-205

[21] Falabella R, Barona MI. Update on skin repigmentation therapies in vitiligo. Pigment Cell Melanoma Res 2009;22:42-65

[22] Khalid M, Mujtaba G. Response of segmental vitiligo to 0.05% clobetasol propionate cream. Int J Dermatol 1998;37:705-8
[23] Silverberg NB, Lin P, Travis L, et al. Tacrolimus ointment promotes repigmentation of vitiligo in children: a review of 57 cases. J Am Acad Dermatol 2004;51:760-6
[24] Udompataikul M, Boonsupthip P, Siriwattanagate R. Effectiveness of 0.1% topical tacrolimus in adult and children patients with vitiligo. J Dermatol 2011;38:536-40
[25] Anbar TS, Westerhof W, Abdel-Rahman AT, et al. Evaluation of the effects of NB-UVB in both segmental and non-segmental vitiligo affecting different body sites. Photodermatol Photoimmunol Photomed 2006;22:157-163
[26] Lotti TM, Menchini G, Andreassi L. UV-B radiation microphototherapy. An elective treatment for segmental vitiligo. J Eur Acad Dermatol Venereol. 1999;13:102-8
[27] Tallab T, Joharji H, Bahamdan K, et al. Response of vitiligo to PUVA therapy in Saudi patients. Int J Dermatol 2005;44:556-558
[28] Spencer JM, Nossa R, Ajmeri J. Treatment of vitiligo with the 308-nm excimer laser: a pilot study. J Am Acad Dermatol 2002;46:727–731
[29] Nicolaidou E, Antoniou C, Stratigos A, et al. Narrowband ultraviolet B phototherapy and 308-nm excimer laser in the treatment of vitiligo: a review. J Am Acad Dermatol 2009;60:470-477
[30] Do JE, Shin JY, Kim DY, et al. The effect of 308nm excimer laser on segmental vitiligo: a retrospective study of 80 patients with segmental vitiligo. Photodermatol Photoimmunol Photomed 2011;27:147-151
[31] Lee DY, Park JH, Lee JH, et al. Surgical treatment is indicated in long-duration segmental vitiligo. Dermatol Surg 2010;36:568-9
[32] Fai D, Cassano N, Vena GA. Narrow-band UVB phototherapy combined with tacrolimus ointment in vitiligo: a review of 110 patients. J Eur Acad Dermatol Venereol. 2007;21:916-20
[33] Lee DY, Kim CR, Lee JH. Targeted phototherapy in combination with drug therapy for segmental vitiligo. Photodermatol Photoimmunol Photomed 2011;27:108-110
[34] Kim CR, Lee DY. Combination of narrow band UVB and topical tacrolimus is effective for segmental vitiligo 2011 Int J Dermatol in press
[35] Yu HS, Wu CS, Yu CL, et al. Helium-neon laser irradiation stimulates migration and proliferation in melanocytes and induces repigmentation in segmental-type vitiligo. J Invest Dermatol 2003;120:56-64
[36] Parsad D, Gupta S; IADVL Dermatosurgery Task Force. Standard guidelines of care for vitiligo surgery. Indian J Dermatol Venereol Leprol. 2008;74 Suppl:S37-45.
[37] Gupta S, Kumar B. Epidermal grafting in vitiligo: influence of age, site of lesion, and type of disease on outcome. J Am Acad Dermatol 2003;49:99-104
[38] Lee KJ, Choi YL, Kim JA, et al. Combination therapy of epidermal graft and systemic corticosteroid for vitiligo. Dermatol Surg 2007;33:1002-1003
[39] Lee DY, Lee KJ, Choi SC, et al. Segmental vitiligo treated by the combination of epidermal grafting and systemic corticosteroids. Dermatol Surg 2010;36:575-576
[40] Lee DY, Park JH, Lee JH, et al. Recurrence of segmental vitiligo after epidermal grafting does not involve epidermal grafting area. Clin Exp Dermatol 2010;35:205-6

8

Vitamin D and Vitiligo

Sang Ho Oh and Miri Kim
Department of Dermatology & Cutaneous Biology Research Institute
Yonsei University College of Medicine, Seoul
Korea

1. Introduction

Vitamin D is a steroid hormone with such pleiotropic effects as bone and calcium homeostasis, as well as immunomodulation, and it exerts its effects via the vitamin D receptor (VDR). Vitamin D can be obtained from food as vitamin D_3 (cholecalciferol), but is also synthesized in the keratinocytes in the epidermis from the precursor molecule 7-dehydrocholesterol (provitamin D3) by ultraviolet B (UVB) radiation in sunlight to pre-vitamin D3. Pre-vitamin D_3 then undergoes a spontaneous, temperature-dependent isomerization to vitamin D_3 (cholecalciferol), which enters the dermal capillaries. At this point, endogenous vitamin D_3 and exogenous dietary D_2 (ergocalciferol) undergo hydroxylation in the liver to 25-hydroxy Vitamin D (calcitriol). This molecule travels to the kidney where it is again hydroxylated to make mature vitamin D (1,25-dihydroxy Vitamin D, or $1,25(OH)_2D_3$, which is also known as calcitriol) and 24,25-dihydroxyvitamin D. $1,25(OH)_2D_3$ is the biologically active form of vitamin D, which regulates serum calcium and phosphate homeostasis.(Klaus Wolff 2008) Circulating $1,25(OH)_2D_3$ has a very short half-life and is tightly regulated by parathyroid hormone. Fibroblast growth factor 23 (FGF23), which is produced in osteoblasts, is also important in regulating $1,25(OH)_2D_3$ production in the kidney.(Jurutka, Bartik et al. 2007)

2. Vitamin D and autoimmune diseases

There is increasing evidence that vitamin D may have an immunoregulatory role in various autoimmune diseases. The mechanism by which vitamin D affects autoimmunity is unknown, but there is clear evidence of regulation of immune cells by vitamin D *in vitro*.(Adorini and Penna 2008; Cantorna, Yu et al. 2008) Vitamin D has multiple effects on innate and adaptive immune responses through its effects on T and B lymphocytes, macrophages, and dendritic cells (DC), all of which express the VDR.(Adorini and Penna 2008) High levels of $1,25(OH)_2D_3$ inhibit dendritic cell maturation with lower expression of major histocompatibility complex (MHC) class II molecules, downregulation of costimulatory molecules that are required for antigen presentation, and lower production of proinflammatory cytokines such as interleukin (IL)-12.(van Etten and Mathieu 2005; Baeke, van Etten et al. 2008) In mouse models, $1,25(OH)_2D_3$ drives the adaptive immune system from a T helper T_h1/T_h17 response toward a T_h2 and regulatory T-cell response, suggesting the potential beneficial effects of vitamin D on the inhibition of T_h1-mediated autoimmune diseases in humans.(Daniel, Sartory et al. 2008) The immune system of VDR-deficient mice is grossly normal but shows increased susceptibility to autoimmune diseases such as inflammatory bowel disease and type 1 diabetes mellitus.(Bouillon, Carmeliet et al. 2008) In addition, $1,25(OH)_2D_3$ may suppress autoimmune diseases by enhancing the production and function of regulatory T cells (Tregs), which are vital for preserving peripheral self-tolerance. $1,25(OH)_2D_3$ plays a role in the activation of Tregs by DCs, by increasing the number of Tregs, and enhancing their secretion of IL-10, which inhibits the activation of T lymphocytes.(Loser, Mehling et al. 2006; Spach, Nashold et al. 2006) There is some evidence that vitamin D may play a regulatory role in autoantibody production by B cells, inhibiting the ongoing proliferation of activated B cells and inducing their apoptosis.(Chen, Sims et al. 2007) Several mechanisms have been proposed to explain the role for vitamin D insufficiency in the pathogenesis of autoimmune disorders.

There are also various reports of vitamin D deficiency associated with several autoimmune disorders, including inflammatory bowel disease, multiple sclerosis (MS), systemic lupus erythematosus (SLE), type 1 diabetes mellitus, and rheumatoid arthritis (RA).(Cantorna, Yu et al. 2008) Furthermore, vitamin D polymorphisms have also been associated with increased risk of multiple autoimmune diseases, including Hashimoto's thyroiditis, inflammatory bowel disease, Graves' disease, rheumatoid arthritis, SLE, primary biliary cirrhosis (PBC), autoimmune hepatitis, Addison's disease, vitiligo, celiac disease, type I diabetes mellitus and multiple sclerosis (MS).(Kriegel, Manson et al. 2011) Therefore, supplementation of vitamin D can possibly be used as a treatment in autoimmune disease. Vitamin D supplementation has been shown to be therapeutically effective in different experimental animal models, such as allergic encephalomyelitis, collagen-induced arthritis, type 1 diabetes mellitus, inflammatory bowel disease, autoimmune thyroiditis, and systemic lupus erythematosus.(Lemire and Archer 1991; Mathieu, Waer et al. 1994; Cantorna, Hayes et al. 1998; Cantorna, Munsick et al. 2000; Van Etten, Branisteanu et al. 2003) However, despite the *in vitro* and animal evidence for the promising effects of vitamin D to decrease systemic inflammation and prevent autoimmune disease in humans, these findings have been somewhat conflicting in humans.

3. Association between vitamin D and vitiligo

Vitiligo, an autoimmune pigmentary disorder, is characterized by the aberrant loss of functional melanocytes from involved epidermis. The association of vitiligo with autoimmune conditions is well-established. Vitiligo is commonly associated with thyroid disorders and abnormalities, particularly Hashimoto's thyroiditis and Grave's disease, type I diabetes mellitus, and Sjögren's syndrome.(Sehgal, Rege et al. 1976; Niepomniszcze and Amad 2001; Montes, Pfister et al. 2003; Adorini and Penna 2008) Low levels of vitamin D have also been associated with autoimmune diseases, including rheumatoid arthritis, type I diabetes mellitus, and multiple sclerosis.(Adorini and Penna 2008) However, little is known about the association of vitiligo and reduced vitamin D levels.

Silverberg *et al.* reported that patients with vitiligo who have low levels of vitamin D were at higher risk for secondary forms of autoimmunity and that insufficient vitamin D levels were associated with increasing Fitzpatrick phototype.(Silverberg, Silverberg et al. 2010) They suggested that monitoring vitamin D levels in patients with vitiligo may identify individuals at greater risk for secondary autoimmune diatheses. However, there is no reliable evidence that vitamin D supplementation can treat or prevent vitiligo.

4. Effect of topical vitamin D on vitiligo

In recent years, topical vitamin D analogues, particularly calcipotriol and tacalcitol, have been used as monotherapy or in combination with phototherapy for the treatment of vitiligo. Even if their exact mechanism of actions were unclear, vitamin D analogues have two different effects on vitiligo in terms of immune function and melanocytes. Vitamin D ligands are designed to target the local immune response in vitiligo, acting specifically on T cell activation, mainly by inhibiting the transition of T cells from the early-to-late G_1 period in interphase and by inhibiting the expression of several pro-inflammatory cytokines genes, such as those encoding tumor necrosis factor-alpha (TNF-α) and interferon gamma (IFN-γ). Vitamin D_3 compounds are known to influence melanocyte maturation and differentiation and also to up-regulate melanogenesis through pathways activated by specific ligand receptors, such as the endothelin receptor and the proto-oncogene c-kit (mast/stem cell growth factor receptor [SCFR]).(Birlea, Costin et al. 2008)

At the molecular level, the addition of vitamin D compounds to a vitiligo treatment regimen along with different forms of UV and glucocorticoids can halt disease progression in vitiligo by immunosuppression and possibly induce repigmentation by activating melanocyte precursors and the promotion of melanogenic pathways.(Birlea, Costin et al. 2009)

However, the true effects of vitamin D analogues on vitiligo remain controversial (Table 1). Some studies have reported a good response or even an augmented response to them over conventional vitiligo therapies, whereas other studies have reported no response to or only limited effects of vitamin D analogues.(Leone, Pacifico et al. 2006; Lu-yan, Wen-wen et al. 2006; Goldinger, Dummer et al. 2007; Rodriguez-Martin, Garcia Bustinduy et al. 2009) One of the authors (SHO) published a prospective study which showed that the use of high concentration tacalcitol had a limited effect as either monotherapy or as part of combination therapy with excimer laser in the treatment of vitiligo.(Oh, Kim et al. 2011)

Treatment	Type of Vitamin D	Study design	Results	Effect	References
Tacalcitol ointment (4μg/g)+ 30min sunlight daily vs placebo + sunlight	Tacalcitol	Randomized, double-blinded, placebo-controlled	Placebo+heliotherapy: 1/31 Tacalcitol+heliotherapy: 0/32 >75% repigmentaton after 4 months	No	(Rodriguez-Martin, Garcia Bustinduy et al. 2009)
NB-UVB vs NB-UVB+ tacalcitol (4μg/g)	Tacalcitol	Randomized, investigator blinded, controlled, left-right trial	NB-UVB: 0/32 NB-UVB+tacalcitol: 16/32 (50%) >80% repigmentation after 6 months	Yes	(Leone, Pacifico et al. 2006)
Excimer light once weekly+ placebo vs excimer light+tacalcitol (2μg/g)	Tacalcitol	Randomized, double-blinded, placebo-controlled, left-right trial	MEL+placebo: 2/35 (5.7%) MEL+tacalcitol: 9/32 (25.7%) >75% repigmentation after 12 treatments (3 months)	Yes	(Lu-yan, Wen-wen et al. 2006)

Treatment	Type of Vitamin D	Study design	Results	Effect	References
Untreated vs calcipotriol	Calcipotriol	Prospective, left/right comparative, open study	3/24: partial response Of 3 patients showing response 1: 5% repigmentation (only treated area) 2: 20% repigmentation (both treated and untreated areas) 3: 30% repigmentation (treated), 10% repigmentation (untreated)	No	(Chiaverini, Passeron et al. 2002)
Betamethasone vs 0.005% calcipotriol vs betamethasone/ calcipotriol	Calcipotriol	Randomized, non-placebo controlled study	All groups: no patients >75% repigmentation Betamethasone: 2/15, Calcipotriol: 1/15, Betamethasone/ calcipotriol: 4/15 50-75% repigmentation Time to repigmentation was faster in combination treatment	No (alone) Yes (combi-nation)	(Kumaran, Kaur et al. 2006)
NB-UVB thrice weekly vs NB-UVB+ calcipotriol (0.05%)	Calcipotriol	Randomized, non-placebo controlled study	NB-UVB: 10/24 (41.67%) NB-UVB + calcipotriol: 6/13 (46.2%) 50-100% repigmentation after 30 treatments (10weeks)	No	(Arca, Tastan et al. 2006)
PUVA+placebo vs PUVA+ calcipotriol (0.05mg/g-0.005%)	Calcipotriol	Randomized, double-blinded, placebo-controlled, left-right trial	PUVA+placebo: 30.07±1.34 treatments PUVA+calcipotriol: 27.4±1.47 treatments (time to complete repigmentation)	Yes	(Ermis, Alpsoy et al. 2001)

Treatment	Type of Vitamin D	Study design	Results	Effect	References
PUVAsol+ placebo vs PUVAsol+calci potriol (50µg/g-0.005%)	Calcipotriol	Randomized, double-blinded, placebo-controlled, left-right trial	PUVAsol+placebo: 9/17 (52.9%) PUVAsol+calcipotriol: 13/17 (76.5%) >75% repigmentation after 18 months	Yes	(Parsad, Saini et al. 1998)
Excimer laser thrice week vs excimer laser +calcipotriol (0.005%)	Calcipotriol	Randomized, single-blinded, left-right trial	Excimer: 22% Excimer +calcipotriol: 23% mean repigmentation after 8 weeks	No	(Goldinger, Dummer et al. 2007)
Excimer laser twice a week vs excimer laser +high concentration of tacalcitol	High concentration of tacalcitol	Randomized, single-blinded, left-right trial	Excimer vs Excimer + tacalcitol: no significant difference	No	(Oh, Kim et al. 2011)

µg/g: microgram/gram, vs: versus, NB-UVB: narrowband ultraviolet B, MEL: monochromatic excimer light, PUVA: psoralen and ultraviolet A, mg/g: milligram/ gram, PUVAsol: psoralen and sun exposure

Table 1. Randomized, controlled studies regarding the effect of vitamin D on the treatment of vitiligo

Vitamin D analogues as monotherapy are less effective than topical corticosteroids in vitiligo, although there is some evidence of an additive effect with combining the two. (Hossani-Madani and Halder 2011) There is no convincing evidence to suggest that topical vitamin D analogues in combination with phototherapy, *i.e.*, narrowband UVB (NB-UVB), psoralen and ultraviolet A (PUVA), or 308 nanometer (nm) excimer laser, are superior to phototherapy alone. Gawkrodger *et al.* recommended that topical vitamin D analogues in combination with NB-UVB or PUVA therapy should not be used in the treatment of vitiligo.(Gawkrodger, Ormerod et al. 2008)

5. Conclusion

Vitiligo is generally considered to be an autoimmune disorder. There is preliminary evidence that vitamin D deficiency could be causally related to a variety of autoimmune diseases. There have been some reports showing good responses to topical vitamin D analogues alone or as part of combination treatment with phototherapy. However, future studies are required to evaluate the relationship of serum vitamin D levels and vitiligo, as well as to elucidate the effects of vitamin D in vitiligo. The utility of topical vitamin D agents in the treatment of vitiligo also needs to be substantiated.

6. References

Adorini, L. and G. Penna (2008). "Control of autoimmune diseases by the vitamin D endocrine system." Nat Clin Pract Rheumatol 4(8): 404-412.

Arca, E., H. B. Tastan, et al. (2006). "Narrow-band ultraviolet B as monotherapy and in combination with topical calcipotriol in the treatment of vitiligo." J Dermatol 33(5): 338-343.

Baeke, F., E. van Etten, et al. (2008). "Vitamin D signaling in immune-mediated disorders: Evolving insights and therapeutic opportunities." Mol Aspects Med 29(6): 376-387.

Birlea, S. A., G. E. Costin, et al. (2008). "Cellular and molecular mechanisms involved in the action of vitamin D analogs targeting vitiligo depigmentation." Curr Drug Targets 9(4): 345-359.

Birlea, S. A., G. E. Costin, et al. (2009). "New insights on therapy with vitamin D analogs targeting the intracellular pathways that control repigmentation in human vitiligo." Med Res Rev 29(3): 514-546.

Bouillon, R., G. Carmeliet, et al. (2008). "Vitamin D and human health: lessons from vitamin D receptor null mice." Endocr Rev 29(6): 726-776.

Cantorna, M. T., C. E. Hayes, et al. (1998). "1,25-Dihydroxycholecalciferol inhibits the progression of arthritis in murine models of human arthritis." J Nutr 128(1): 68-72.

Cantorna, M. T., C. Munsick, et al. (2000). "1,25-Dihydroxycholecalciferol prevents and ameliorates symptoms of experimental murine inflammatory bowel disease." J Nutr 130(11): 2648-2652.

Cantorna, M. T., S. Yu, et al. (2008). "The paradoxical effects of vitamin D on type 1 mediated immunity." Mol Aspects Med 29(6): 369-375.

Chen, S., G. P. Sims, et al. (2007). "Modulatory effects of 1,25-dihydroxyvitamin D3 on human B cell differentiation." J Immunol 179(3): 1634-1647.

Chiaverini, C., T. Passeron, et al. (2002). "Treatment of vitiligo by topical calcipotriol." J Eur Acad Dermatol Venereol 16(2): 137-138.

Daniel, C., N. A. Sartory, et al. (2008). "Immune modulatory treatment of trinitrobenzene sulfonic acid colitis with calcitriol is associated with a change of a T helper (Th) 1/Th17 to a Th2 and regulatory T cell profile." J Pharmacol Exp Ther 324(1): 23-33.

Ermis, O., E. Alpsoy, et al. (2001). "Is the efficacy of psoralen plus ultraviolet A therapy for vitiligo enhanced by concurrent topical calcipotriol? A placebo-controlled double-blind study." Br J Dermatol 145(3): 472-475.

Gawkrodger, D. J., A. D. Ormerod, et al. (2008). "Guideline for the diagnosis and management of vitiligo." Br J Dermatol 159(5): 1051-1076.

Goldinger, S. M., R. Dummer, et al. (2007). "Combination of 308-nm xenon chloride excimer laser and topical calcipotriol in vitiligo." J Eur Acad Dermatol Venereol 21(4): 504-508.

Hossani-Madani, A. and R. Halder (2011). "Treatment of vitiligo: advantages and disadvantages, indications for use and outcomes." G Ital Dermatol Venereol 146(5): 373-395.

Jurutka, P. W., L. Bartik, et al. (2007). "Vitamin D receptor: key roles in bone mineral pathophysiology, molecular mechanism of action, and novel nutritional ligands." J Bone Miner Res 22 Suppl 2: V2-10.

Klaus Wolff, L. G., Stephen Katz, Barbara A. Gilchrest, Barbara Gilchrest, Amy Paller, David J. Leffell, David Leffell (2008). Fitzpatrick's Dermatology in General Medicine. New York, McGraw-Hill Medical.

Kriegel, M. A., J. E. Manson, et al. (2011). "Does vitamin D affect risk of developing autoimmune disease?: a systematic review." Semin Arthritis Rheum 40(6): 512-531 e518.

Kumaran, M. S., I. Kaur, et al. (2006). "Effect of topical calcipotriol, betamethasone dipropionate and their combination in the treatment of localized vitiligo." J Eur Acad Dermatol Venereol 20(3): 269-273.

Lemire, J. M. and D. C. Archer (1991). "1,25-dihydroxyvitamin D3 prevents the in vivo induction of murine experimental autoimmune encephalomyelitis." J Clin Invest 87(3): 1103-1107.

Leone, G., A. Pacifico, et al. (2006). "Tacalcitol and narrow-band phototherapy in patients with vitiligo." Clin Exp Dermatol 31(2): 200-205.

Loser, K., A. Mehling, et al. (2006). "Epidermal RANKL controls regulatory T-cell numbers via activation of dendritic cells." Nat Med 12(12): 1372-1379.

Lu-yan, T., F. Wen-wen, et al. (2006). "Topical tacalcitol and 308-nm monochromatic excimer light: a synergistic combination for the treatment of vitiligo." Photodermatol Photoimmunol Photomed 22(6): 310-314.

Mathieu, C., M. Waer, et al. (1994). "Prevention of autoimmune diabetes in NOD mice by 1,25 dihydroxyvitamin D3." Diabetologia 37(6): 552-558.

Montes, L. F., R. Pfister, et al. (2003). "Association of vitiligo with Sjogren's syndrome." Acta Derm Venereol 83(4): 293.

Niepomniszcze, H. and R. H. Amad (2001). "Skin disorders and thyroid diseases." J Endocrinol Invest 24(8): 628-638.

Oh, S. H., T. Kim, et al. (2011). "Combination treatment of non-segmental vitiligo with a 308-nm xenon chloride excimer laser and topical high-concentration tacalcitol: a prospective, single-blinded, paired, comparative study." J Am Acad Dermatol 65(2): 428-430.

Parsad, D., R. Saini, et al. (1998). "Combination of PUVAsol and topical calcipotriol in vitiligo." Dermatology 197(2): 167-170.

Rodriguez-Martin, M., M. Garcia Bustinduy, et al. (2009). "Randomized, double-blind clinical trial to evaluate the efficacy of topical tacalcitol and sunlight exposure in the treatment of adult nonsegmental vitiligo." Br J Dermatol 160(2): 409-414.

Sehgal, V. N., V. L. Rege, et al. (1976). "Clinical pattern of vitiligo amongst Indians." The Journal of dermatology 3(2): 49-53.

Silverberg, J. I., A. I. Silverberg, et al. (2010). "A pilot study assessing the role of 25 hydroxy vitamin D levels in patients with vitiligo vulgaris." J Am Acad Dermatol 62(6): 937-941.

Spach, K. M., F. E. Nashold, et al. (2006). "IL-10 signaling is essential for 1,25-dihydroxyvitamin D3-mediated inhibition of experimental autoimmune encephalomyelitis." J Immunol 177(9): 6030-6037.

Van Etten, E., D. D. Branisteanu, et al. (2003). "Combination of a 1,25-dihydroxyvitamin D3 analog and a bisphosphonate prevents experimental autoimmune encephalomyelitis and preserves bone." Bone 32(4): 397-404.

van Etten, E. and C. Mathieu (2005). "Immunoregulation by 1,25-dihydroxyvitamin D3: basic concepts." J Steroid Biochem Mol Biol 97(1-2): 93-101.

9

Topical Calcineurin Inhibitors in the Treatment of Vitiligo

Cristina Caridi, Andrew Sohn and Rita V. Patel
Department of Dermatology, Mount Sinai School of Medicine, New York
USA

1. Introduction

Vitiligo is the most common depigmenting disorder, with a prevalence of approximately 0.5% in the world population. Almost half of the patients with vitiligo present before 20 years of age. The two sexes are affected equally, and there are no apparent differences according to skin type or race.[1,2] On histology, vitiligo is identified by the loss of epidermal melanocytes with absence of inflammation.

Commonly used repigmentation therapies whose efficacy is supported by data from randomized controlled trials include ultraviolet light (for whole body or targeted lesions) and topical agents (corticosteroids and calcineurin inhibitors). Narrow-band ultraviolet B radiation (NB-UVB), which delivers peak emission at 311nm, is currently the preferred treatment for adults and children with vitiligo. Topical therapies may be effective in cases of localized disease. Combination therapy is often considered when there has been no response to phototherapy alone after three months or when the goal is to accelerate the response and reduce cumulative exposure to UV light.[3] This chapter will review the literature on the topical use of pimecrolimus and tacrolimus in the treatment of vitiligo alone as well as when combined with other common therapies.

2. Pimecrolimus

Topical calcineurin inhibitors have shown promise in the repigmentation of affected areas in patients with vitiligo without causing the adverse effect profile associated with other common treatments for this disease.[4] Pimecrolimus has been approved for the treatment of atopic dermatitis and has shown a very low incidence of side effects In comparison, corticosteroids can cause thinning of the skin as well as epidermal atrophy at the application site, and PUVA has an associated skin cancer risk.[5] Thus far, pimecrolimus has shown a very low incidence of mild, temporary adverse effects including erythema and irritation at the application site,[6] which makes this modality a safe treatment option. It appears that pimecrolimus may offer a considerable advantage in cases where the side effects of other therapies are of greater concern as in vitiligo occurring in pediatric patients or disease affecting facial, intertriginous, and genital regions, as neither epidermal atrophy nor telangiectasia are major concerns.[2]

There are several hypotheses about the pathogenesis of vitiligo, but there is increased evidence of an auto-immune mechanism involving both humoral and cellular immunity.

This has been supported by the frequent detection of circulating auto-antibodies, cytoplasmatic antigens of melanocytes, and activated T-cells in the periphery of actively progressing lesions in vitiligo patients.[7] An analysis of 19 vitiligo patients for 24 weeks showed that, at baseline, patients expressed a significant increase in the expression of interferon-γ, tumor necrosis factor alpha (TNF-α) expression, and IL-10 in involved and uninvolved skin as compared to healthy patients. After treatment, TNF-α expression decreased in involved and adjacent uninvolved skin, illustrating a relationship between cytokine imbalance and the depigmentation process of vitiligo.[8]

Pimecrolimus inhibits the production of T-cells and prevents mast cells from releasing pro-inflammatory mediators.[9] The structure of pimecrolimus has higher lipophilicity than that of tacrolimus and binds to macrophilin 12 with high affinity.[10] This complex inhibits calcineurin resulting in the suppression of pro-inflammatory cytokine[1] secretion by activated T-cells, specifically that of interferon-γ, IL-1, IL-2, IL-3, IL-4, IL-5, GM-CSF, and TNF-α[11,12] which are believed to be responsible for the damage to melanocytes that results in vitiligo. *In vitro* research on the effect of calcineurin inhibitors on melanocytes affected by vitiligo may further support the hypothesis that the pathogenesis of vitiligo involves an auto-immune response as well as autocytotoxic components. It has been observed *in vitro* that the interaction between calcineurin inhibitors and keratinocytes induces the release of stem cell factor and enhancing matrix metalloproteinase-9 activity, allowing melanocytes to grow.[13]

A study evaluating the efficacy of topical 0.05% clobetasol propionate versus 1% pimecrolimus ointment indicated that pimecrolimus is just as effective as clobetasol propionate in repigmenting skin without producing the side effects that often result in the discontinuation of steroid treatment. The study group included 10 patients ranging in age from 12-66 years old with generalized vitiligo ranging in duration from two to 40 years. Affected regions varied from extremities, trunk, or acral regions. There was no statistically significant difference in the degree of repigmentation resulting from pimecrolimus versus clobetasol propionate, but atrophy and telangiectasia were reported in the clobetasol propionate treatment group, indicating that pimecrolimus has a more favorable safety profile than clobetasol. Two patients being treated with pimecrolimus reported experiencing a mild burning sensation that was not severe enough to result in the discontinuation of treatment.[14] Topical corticosteroids are indicated in the treatment of vitiligo and have been a common treatment for approximately 30 years.[15] Recurrence of symptoms of vitiligo and the relatively high incidence of adverse effects including atrophy, telangiectasia, striae, and contact dermatitis are limiting factors particularly for children and sensitive areas of the skin.[10,16]

Because of the low-toxicity of pimecrolimus, it may be a treatment of particular interest in more sensitive areas affected by vitiligo such as the periocular and genital regions and in pediatric patients. In a case study conducted by Leite et al.[7] an eight-year old patient showed near-complete remission of symptoms of vitiligo in the periocular area after four months of treatment and with no relapse one year thereafter. In another case study presented in Leite et. al. study, an eleven-year-old boy achieved almost complete repigmentation of all vitiligo lesions in the genital region after three months of treatment. Both patients showed good tolerability to the treatment regimen indicating that pimecrolimus may be a safer option for the skin of children and adolescents whose skin shows greater predilection for local side-effects.[7]

In a study conducted by Mayoral et al., eight adults presenting with facial vitiligo were treated with pimecrolimus 1% cream twice a day for at least three months. The average length of the study was eleven months from baseline to the final follow-up visit. Patients showed a statistically significant response, averaging 72.5% improvement in pigmentation of the facial region.Every patient showed a response to study treatment regardless of length of disease, extent of disease, or previous treatment regimen, including patients who had not responded to previous therapies including PUVA and Melagenina®. It was observed that the greatest improvement in surface area correlated with the longest duration of disease at baseline and had no significant association with longer treatment duration. Treatment was well tolerated.[8]

The combination of pimecrolimus with other common treatment modalities for vitiligo has been studied to determine whether the degree of response to treatment could be improved or the response time could be accelerated. Esfandiarpour et al. conducted a double-blind, placebo-controlled study to determine the efficacy of pimecrolimus 1% cream combined with NB-UVB in the treatment of vitiligo.[1] NB-UVB has been recently introduced as a similar, safer treatment option than PUVA. Although these photochemotherapy (NB-UVB and PUVA) do have some local immunomodulatory effects, these treatment methods are effective most likely because of the stimulation of melanocyte proliferation.[17,18] It was hypothesized that the addition of pimecrolimus 1% cream to treatment with NB-UVB would better address the autoimmune components of the disease. In this study, 68 patients were randomized into one of two groups: NB-UVB plus pimecrolimus 1% cream or NB-UVB plus placebo for three months. After 12 weeks of treatment, statistically significant repigmentation occurred in more than 50% of facial lesions in 64.3% of patients in the group that received NB-UVB plus pimecrolimus 1% versus 25.1% of patients in the group that received NB-UVB plus placebo. There was no significant difference in the repigmentation rate of other body areas between the two groups.[1]

Another study explored the addition of microdermabrasion in the treatment of nonsegmental vitiligo in children with pimecrolimus 1% cream. It is believed that microdermabrasion may modulate the immune response and autoinoculation of melanocytes as well as enhance the absorption of topical immunomodulators through the inflammation and erosion of the skin. The purpose of this study was to determine if microdermabrasion would be effective in enhancing the efficacy and decreasing the treatment time. Results indicated a positive response to treatment, as 60.4% of lesions treated by combined therapy showed a clinical response, with 43.4% of lesions treated by combined therapy showing complete repigmentation after a three month treatment period, compared with 32.1% repigmentation of lesions treated with pimecrolimus alone, and 1.7% for placebo.[19]

3. Tacrolimus

Topical tacrolimus is a potential therapeutic option for the management of vitiligo. Despite this drug's clinical efficacy, the underlying mechanism of topical tacrolimus in the management of vitiligo is not well understood and has been rarely studied. Tacrolimus is a non-steroidal anti-inflammatory agent used in the treatment and management of many skin disorders and was initially formulated for atopic dermatitis. Similarly to pimecrolimus, tacrolimus exerts its therapeutic effects by targeting and inhibiting calcineurin in the skin, which regulates T-cell division and activation, and in turn inhibits pro-inflammatory cytokines.[20] Systemically administered tacrolimus is an effective immunosuppressant that is used as an anti-rejection agent in organ transplantation, and due to its effective immunosuppression, systemic tacrolimus increases the risk for skin cancer.[21] Topical tacrolimus, however, has not been associated with systemic immunosuppression or increased risk for malignancies in long-term clinical research.[22,23,24] The avoidance of natural and/or artificial light during tacrolimus therapy and application of sunscreen daily is advised.

Multiple studies have documented the stimulatory effects of UV light on melanogenesis and melanocyte proliferation.[25,26] The therapeutic effects of psoralen photochemotherapy and phototherapy with NB-UVB for the repigmentation of vitiliginous skin have also been documented.[27,28] The suppression of pro-inflammatory cytokines via tacrolimus may facilitate the stimulatory effects of ultraviolet light on the repigmentation of vitiliginous skin. Evidence suggests a suppression of TNF-α after application of tacrolimus, which may play a role in repigmentation.[21] TNF-α has been shown to inhibit melanocyte proliferation and melanogenesis, which has allowed for speculation that epidermal cytokines may be a part of a negative feedback that negates the stimulus of melanocytes.[29] Additionally, a number of cytokines, including TNF-α are shown to up-regulate the expression of intercellular adhesion molecule-1 (ICAM-1) on melanocytes, which may trigger a lymphocyte-melanocyte attachment and play a role in the destruction of melanocytes.[30,31] Because tacrolimus inhibits T-cells and therefore cytokines, including TNF-α, tacrolimus may help prevent the aforementioned negative feedback loop as well as the expression of ICAM-1 on melanocytes.

Studies have shown that topical corticosteroids and topical tacrolimus are similarly efficacious in the repigmentation of both facial and nonfacial vitiliginous lesions.[32,33] However, long-term use of topical corticosteroids is contraindicated due to their serious side effects. Therefore, topical tacrolimus offers many advantages over topical corticosteroids for the management of chronic skin disorders including vitiligo. In contrast to topical corticosteroid treatment which results in a predominantly diffuse pattern of repigmentation,[34] topical tacrolimus often induces follicular repigmentation. This indicates the involvement of melanoblast in the repigmentation process, namely the proliferation of inactive melanocytes (melanoblasts), which migrate to the nearby epidermis to differentiate and form perifollicular pigment islands.[35,36,37] Topical tacrolimus induces follicular repigmentation better in sun-exposed anatomical sites. Keratinocytes are known to secrete endothelin, a prodifferentiation factor of melanoblasts, after exposure to UVB radiation.[38] Therefore, sun-exposed keratinocytes most likely provide the necessary endothelin for optimal melanoblast differentiation effect induced by topical tacrolimus.[10]

Topical tacrolimus has been reported to promote melanoblast differentiation and growth. Additionally, topical tacrolimus promotes a favorable environment that fosters the proliferation of melanocytes/melanoblasts through an interaction with keratinocytes, and thereby repopulating vitiliginous skin lesions.[10] In another study by Kang et. al.,[39] topical tacrolimus was seen to induce tyrosinase, which eventually leads to melanin biosynthesis, activity, and expression.

Studies have shown mixed results for combination therapy, consisting of topical tacrolimus and UVB.[40,41,42,43] The use of topical tacrolimus in association with phototherapy gives rise to concern about the possibility of an increased risk to skin malignancies.[44] However, the results of a 2005 study on hairless mice suggest that topical tacrolimus prevents DNA photodamage due to a filter effect of both active and vehicle components in topical formulation but does not affect the clearance of DNA photoproducts.[45] Fai et. al., employed combined therapy, and indicated a rapid and relevant improvement of facial vitiligo, followed by lesions on the limbs and trunk (including the neck), whereas the overall response of vitiligo in other skin areas (extremities and genital areas) was poor.[46] This fact has been attributed to the greater density of hair follicles in the head and neck areas, and thus, greater melanocyte reservoirs.[47] Further long-term efficacy and safety data and randomized controlled trials on a large number of study participants are required.

Combined therapy of topical tacrolimus and 308-nm excimer laser in the management of vitiligo has been evaluated as well. Unlike topical tacrolimus and UVB phototherapy, combination treatment of topical tacrolimus and 308-nm excimer laser has been reported to be more effective and faster than that of excimer laser in monotherapy.[48,49] In comparison with NB-UVB, phototherapy with excimer laser has the advantaged of a targeted treatment, thereby limiting the delivery of radiation only to affected vitiligo skin areas. However, NB-UVB may be more useful for the treatment of extensive vitiligo and is more advantageous than excimer phototherapy with regards to cost, session duration, and patient compliance.[42]

Occlusive treatment has been reported to enhance topical tacrolimus efficacy in treating vitiligo. As mentioned earlier, it has been shown that when applying tacrolimus openly on extremities, there was negligible effect. However, Hartmann et. al.[50] used polyurethane foil or hydrocolloid dressings for overnight occlusive treatment, and moderate to excellent repigmentation was achieved, depending on the dressing utilized. It was suggested that since hydrocolloid dressings lead to higher stratum corneum water holding capacity compared with polyurethane foil[51], the hydrocolloid dressings may be more suitable for enhancing the transcutaneous penetration of the topically applied agent. Moreover, the Hartmann et. al. study had also measured serum concentrations of tacrolimus. All study subjects had tacrolimus serum levels below the detection limit after 12 months, indicating the long-term topical treatment with additional long-term occlusion of areas up to 150 cm^2 does not lead to accumulation of tacrolimus in the blood.[47] Still, larger placebo-controlled studies using topical tacrolimus in combination with occlusion, penetration enhancers, or phototherapy, or in higher concentrations, are required to determine the exact role of topical tacrolimus in the treatment of vitiligo and its optimal mode of use.

4. Conclusion

In conclusion, topical pimecrolimus and tacrolimus are effective and well tolerated treatment options for both adults and children with vitiligo. Moreover, it has been documented that topical tacrolimus has better outcomes for the treatment of vitiligo in children[52] and in patients of skin of color.[53] Topical calcineurin inhibitors are a great alternative for persons with vitiligo but with poor compliance to phototherapy and/or with fear of the side-effects of using topical corticosteroids long-term. Further randomized controlled studies are needed to enhance the understanding of how these topical medications work. Additionally, combination therapy utilizing NB-UVB or eximer laser with topical calcineurin inhibitors should be evaluated in larger trials so that safety and efficacy data can help guide clinicians in managing vilitigo when presented with refractory cases.

5. References

[1] Howitz J, Broadthagen H, Swartz M et al. Prevalence of vitiligo: epidemiolofical survey on the Isle of Bornhold, Denmark. Arch Dermatol 1977; 113: 47-52.

[2] Boisseus-Garsaud AM, Garsaud P, Cales-Quist D et al. Epidemiology of bitiligo in the French West Indes. Int J Dermatol 2000; 39: 18-20.

[3] Taieb A and Picardo M. Vitiligo. New Engl J Med 2009; 360: 160-169.

[4] Esfandiarpour I, Ekhlasi A, Farajzadeh S, Shamsadini S. The efficacy of pimecrolimus 1% cream plus narrow-band ultraviolet B in the treatment of vitiligo: A double-blind, placebo controlled clinical trial. *Journal of Dermatological Treatment*. 2009; 20:1; 14-18.

[5] Sendur N, Karaman G, Sanic N, Savk E. Topical pimecrolimus: A new horizon for vitiligo treatment? *Journal of Dermatological Treatment*. 2006; 17: 338-342.

[6] Ashcroft DM, Dimmock P, Garside R, Stein K, Williams HC. Efficacy and tolerability of topical pimecrolimus and tacrolimus in the treatment of atopic dermatitis: meta-analysis of randomized controlled trials. *BMJ*. 2005 Mar 5;330(7490):516.

[7] Nordlund JJ. The epidemiology and genetics of vitiligo. Clin Dermatol 1997; 15: 875-8

[8] Grimes PE, Morris R, Avaniss-Aghajani E, et al. Topical tacrolimus therapy for vitiligo: therapeutic responses and skin messenger RNA expression of proinflammatory cytokines. *J Am Acad Dermatol* 2004; 51: 52-61.

[9] Dawid M, Veensalu M, Grassberger M, Wolff K. Efficacy and safety of pimecrolimus cream 1% in adult patients with vitiligo: Results of a randomized, double-blind, vehicle-controlled study. *JDDG*;2006 4:942-946.

[10] Billich A, Aschauer H, Aszodi A, Stuetz A. Percutaneous absorption of drugs used in atopic eczema: pimecrolimus permeates less through skin than corticosteroids and tacrolimus. *International Journal of Pharmaceutics*. 2004; 269:29-35.

[11] Seifari H, Farnaghi F, Firooz A, Vasheghani-Farahani A, Alirezaie N-S, Dowlati Y. Pimecrolimus cream in repigmentation of vitiligo. *Dermatology*. 2007;214:253-259.

[12] Mayoral FA, Vega JM, Stavisky H, McCormick CL, Parneix-Spake A. Retrospective analysis of pimecrolimus cream 1% for treatment of facial vitiligo. *J Drugs Dermatol*. 2007 May;6(5):517-21.

[13] Lan CCE, Chen GS, Chiou MH, Wu CS. FK506 promotes melanocyte and melanoblast growth and creates a favourable milieu for cell migration via keratinocytes: possible mechanisms of how tacrolimus ointment induces repigmentation in patients with vitiligo. *Br J Dermatol*. 2005; 153:498-505.

[14] Coskun B, Saral Y, Turgut D. Topical 0.05% clobetosol propionate versus 1% pimecrolimus ointment in vitiligo. *Eur J Dermatol* 2005 Mar-Apr;15(2):88-91.

[15] Mosher DB, Fitzpatrick TB, Ortonne JP, Hori Y. Hypomelanoses and hypermelanoses. In: Freedberg IM, Eisen AZ, Wolff K, et. al., eds. *Dermatology in General Medicine*. 5th ed. New York: McGraw Hill, 1999: 949-60.

[16] Kostovic K, Nola I, Bucan Z, Situm M. Treatment of vitiligo: current methods and new approaches. *Acta Dermatovenerol Croat* 2003; 11:1633-70.

[17] Borderé AC, Lambert J, van Geel N. Current and emerging therapy for the management of vitiligo. *Clin Cosmet Investig Dermatol*. 2009; 2: 15-25.

[18] Fitzpatrick TB. Mechanisms of phototherapy of vitiligo. *Arch Dermatol*. 1997 Dec;133(12):1525-8.

[19] Farajzadeh S, Daraei Z, Esfandiarpour I, Hosseini SH. The efficacy of Pimecrolimus 1% cream combined with microdermabrasion in the treatment of nonsegmental

childhood vitiligo: a randomized placebo-controlled study. *Pedictric Dermatology* 2009 May-Jun;26(3):286-91.
[20] Nghiem P, Pearson G, Langley RG. Tacrolimus and pimecrolimus: From clever prokaryotes to inhibiting calcineurin and treating atopic dermatitis. *J Am Acad Dermatol.* 2002; 46:228-41.
[21] Woodle ES, Thistlethwaite JR, Gordon JH, Laskow D, Deierhoi MH, Burdick J, et al. A multicenter trial of FK506 (tacrolimus) therapy in refractory acute renal allograft rejection. A report of the Tacrolimus Kidney Transplantation Rescue, Study Group. Transplantation 1996;62:594-9.
[22] Kang S, Lucky AW, Pariser D, Lawrence I, Hanifin JM, Tacrolimus Ointment Study Group. Long-term safety and efficacy of tacrolimus ointment for the treatment of atopic dermatitis in children. J Am Acad Dermatol 2001;44:S58-64.
[23] Paller AS, Caro I, Rico MJ, and the Tacrolimus Ointment Study Group. Long-term safety and efficacy of tacrolimus ointment monotherapy in atopic dermatitis patients: open-label study results. Ann Dermatol Venereol 2002;129(Suppl 1):S247.
[24] Koo JYM, Prose N, Fleischer A, Rico MJ, Tacrolimus Ointment Study Group. Safety and efficacy of tacrolimus ointment monotherapy in over 7900 atopic dermatitis patients: results of an open-label study. Ann Dermatol Venereol 2002; 129(Suppl 1):S415.
[25] Jimbow K, Uesugi T. New melanogenesis and photobiological processes in activation and proliferation of precursor melanocytes after UV-exposure ultrastructural differentiation of precursor melanocytes from Langerhans cells. J Invest Dermatol 1982;78:108-15.
[26] Friedmann PS, Gilchrest BA. Ultraviolet radiation directly induces pigment production by cultured human melanocytes. J Cell Physiol13321198788-94.
[27] Grimes PE. Vitiligo an overview of therapeutic approaches. Dermatol Clin 1993;11:325-38.
[28] Grimes PE. Therapeutic trends for the treatment of vitiligo. Cosmetic Dermatol 2002;15:21-5.
[29] Swope VB, Abdel-Malek Z, Kassem LM, Nordlund JJ. Interleukins 1a and 6 and tumor necrosis factor-a are paracrine inhibitors of human melanocyte proliferation and melanogenesis. J Invest Dermatol 1991;96:180-5.
[30] Yohn JJ, Critelli M, Lyons MB, Norris DA. Modulation of melanocyte intercellular adhesion molecule-1 by immune cytokines. J Invest Dermatol 1990;90:233-7.
[31] Morelli JG, Norris DA. Influence of inflammatory mediators and cytokines on human melanocyte function. J Invest Dermatol 1993;100(Suppl):191S-5S.
[32] Ho N, Pope E, Weinstein M, et. al. A double-blind, randomized, placebo-controlled trial of topical tacrolimus 0·1% vs.clobetasol propionate 0·05% in childhood vitiligo. Br J Dermatol 2011; doi: 10.1111/ j.13652133. 2011. 10351.x [Epub ahead of print].
[33] Lepe V, Moncada B, Castanedo-Cazares JP, et. al. A double-blind randomized trial of 0.1% tacrolimus vs 0.05% clobetasol for the treatment of childhood vitiligo. Arch Dermatol 2003;139(5):581-5.
[34] Parsad D, Pandhi R, Dogra S, Kumar B. Clinical study of repigmentation patterns with different treatment modalities and their correlation with speed and stability of repigmentation in 352 vitiliginous patches. J Am Acad Dermatol 2004; 50:63–7.
[35] Silverberg NB, Lin P, Travis L et al. Tacrolimus ointment promotes repigmentation of vitiligo in children: a review of 57 cases. J Am Acad Dermatol 2004; 51:760–6.

[36] Kenwar AJ, Dogra S, Parsad D. Topical tacrolimus for treatment of childhood vitiligo in Asians. Clin Exp Dermatol 2004; 29:589–92.

[37] Fitzpatrick TB. Mechanisms of photochemotherapy of vitiligo. Arch Dermatol 1997; 133:1591–2.

[38] Imokawa G, Miyagishi M, Yada Y. Endothelin-1 as a new melanogen: coordinated expression of its gene and the tyrosinase gene in UVB-exposed human epidermis. J Invest Dermatol 1995; 105:32–7.

[39] Kang HY, Choi YM. FK506 increases pigmentation and migration of human melanocytes. Br J Dermatol 2006; 155(5):1037-40.

[40] Castanedo-Cazares JP, Lepe V, Moncada B. Repigmentation of chronic vitiligo lesions by following tacrolimus plus ultraviolet-B-narrow-band. *Photodermatol Photoimmunol Photomed* 2003; 19:35–36.

[41] Mehrabi D, Pandya AG. A randomized, placebo-controlled, double-blind trial comparing narrow-band UV-B Plus 0.1% tacrolimus ointment with narrow-band UV-B plus placebo in the treatment of generalized vitiligo. *Arch Dermatol* 2006; 142:927–929.

[42] Stinco G, Piccirillo F, Forcione M, et. al. An open randomized study to compare narrow band UVB, topical pimecrolimus and topical tacrolimus in the treatment of vitiligo. Eur J Dermatol 2009; 19(6):588-93.

[43] Nordal E, Guleng G, Ronneviq J. Treatment of vitiligo with narrowband-UVB (TL01) combined with tacrolimus ointment (0.1%) vs. placebo ointment, a randomized right/left double-blind comparative study.

[44] Yarosh DB, Pena AV, Nay SL *et al.* Calcineurin inhibitors decrease DNA repair and apoptosis in human keratinocytes following ultraviolet B irradiation. *J Invest Dermatol* 2005; 125: 1020–1025.

[45] Tran C, Lubbe J, Sorg O *et al.* Topical calcineurin inhibitors decrease the production of UVB-induced thymine dimmers from hairless mouse epidermis. *Dermatology* 2005; 211: 341–347.

[46] Tran C, Lubbe J, Sorg O *et al.* Topical calcineurin inhibitors decrease the production of UVB-induced thymine dimmers from hairless mouse epidermis. *Dermatology* 2005; 211: 341–347.

[47] Cui J, Shen LY, Wang GC. Role of hair follicles in the repigmentation of vitiligo. J Invest Dermatol 1991; 97:410–416.

[48] Kawalek AZ, Spencer JM, Phelps RG. Combined excimer laser and topical tacrolimus for the treatment of vitiligo: a pilot study. *Dermatol Surg* 2004; 30: 130–135.

[49] Passeron T, Ostovari N, Zakaria W *et al.* Topical tacrolimus and the 308-nm excimer laser: a synergistic combination for the treatment of vitiligo. *Arch Dermatol* 2004; 140:1065–1069.

[50] Hartmann A, Brocker EB, Hamm H. Occlusive treatment enhances efficacy of tacrolimus 0.1% ointment in adult patients with vitiligo: results of a placebo-controlled 12-month prospective study. Acta Derm Venereol 2008; 88(5):474-9.

[51] Berardesca E, Vignoli GP, Fideli D, Maibach H. Effect of occlusive dressings on the stratum corneum water holding capacity. Am J Med Sci 1992; 304:25-28.

[52] Udompataikul M, Boonsupthip P, Siriwattanagate R. Effectiveness of 0.1% topical tacrolimus in adult and children patients with vitiligo. J Dermatol. 2011; 38(6):536-40. doi: 10.1111/j.1346-8138.2010.01067.x. Epub 2010 Nov 2.

[53] Silverberg JI, Silverberg NB. Topical tacrolimus is more effective for treatment of vitiligo in patients of skin of color. J Drugs Dermatol. 2011; 10(5):507-10.

10

Complementary and Alternative Medicine for Vitiligo

Jimi Yoon[1], Young-Woo Sun[2] and Tae-Heung Kim[2]
[1]*Gyeongsang National University Hospital*
[2]*White-Line Skin Clinic & Research Center, Kyungnam*
Republic of Korea

1. Introduction

We are in an era of modern medicine that is defined by rapid change. Scientists are accumulating and analyzing scores of genomic data, however, the majority of data being accumulated on vitiligo has not been appropriately archived or systemized for analysis (Alikhan *et al*, 2011; Spritz, 2011).

The pathogenensis of vitiligo is multifactorial, and includes three main factors: genetic, immunological, and environmental. Clinically, environmental factors are important in the development of vitiligo. Trauma, eczema, chemical agents, and fragility of keratinocytes play a role in development of vitiligo, so treatment decisions should be made taking these factors into account (Alikhan *et al*, 2011; Lee *et al*, 2005).

Historically, vitiligo was deemed to respond relatively poorly to treatment with a high recurrence rate, therefore, there is at times a reluctance to advise treatment. Recently, various treatment modalities have been introduced, and treatment options and outcomes have been improving. Excimer laser, phototherapy, epidermal grafts, and lifestyle modification have improved the results of treatment and quality of lives of patients with vitiligo (Felsten *et al*, 2011).

South Korea is a country (approximately 1/7th the size of Texas) with excellent modern medical facilities for the treatment of vitiligo. There are 130 practices where eximer lasers are commonly used and more than 70 practices can provide surgical management (epidermal grafts). Nevertheless, many patients seek alternative medical options, including oriental medicines and folk remedies for treatment of their vitiligo. Dermatologists should have an objective point of view on how to use and combine complementary and alternative medicine (CAM) with modern medicine. This chapter will review the various complementary and alternative medicines and evaluate their efficacy and safety to validate their reliability.

2. Vitiligo and lifestyle modification

The location of vitiligo can give clues as to its triggers or causes. In stress-induced cases, skin lesions are frequently localized to the seborrheic area (Figure 1A). In traumatic types, the lesions are usually localized to sites of injury or pressure (Figure 1B). In dermatitis-associated types, depigmented lesions tend to occur in areas of a specific pre-existing dermatitis. Doctors can often assume predisposing and aggravating factors that can help identify vitiligo etiology, and thereby advise patients to alter modifiable living habits (Taïeb & Picardo, 2009).

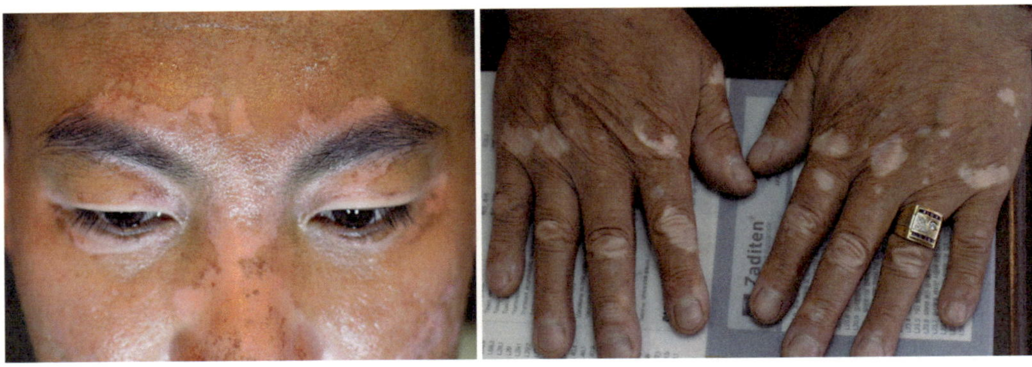

Fig. 1. A. Vitiligo in a seborrheic distribution. B. Vitiligo on the bony prominences.

2.1 Diet, food additives, antioxidants, vitamins, and microelements

Diet is not considered very important in the treatment of vitiligo. However, a healthy, balanced diet with nutrients from a variety of sources can be helpful in vitiligo. According to complementary and alternative medicine (CAM) practitioners, there are foods that are considered either beneficial for or detrimental in vitiligo, but they differ in opinion about these foods and they often lack medical evidence to substantiate their claims. Often, recommendations are determined by a food's composition of antioxidants, vitamins, and microelements. On the other hand, the detrimental effects of foods or food additives are often based on the risk of allergic reactions and irritation, either of which could trigger or exacerbate vitiligo.

2.1.1 What foods should be avoided?

Some Ayurvedic specialists insist that certain foods are harmful to the body when a patient is suffering from vitiligo. This includes tamarind, tomatoes, citrus fruits and juices, grapes, papayas, sour or pickled food items, tinned foods or drinks, chocolate and cocoa products, coffee, oily or spicy foods, blueberries, pears, eggs, dairy products, and fish (Ravish, 2011). Traditional Korean medicine specialists do not recommend consuming pork, chicken, and wheat for patients with vitiligo. There are also homeopathic doctors who suggest that sour foods, ascorbic acid, non-vegetarian foods, and flavored drinks and foods with artificial colors may worsen the condition.

Namazi & Chee Leok (2009) suggested that mangoes, cashews, pistachios, oak, cassavas, areca nuts, red chilies, cherries, raspberries, cranberries, blackberries, and tea contain naturally-occurring plant phenols and polyphenolic compounds, or tannins, that could possibly aggravate vitiligo due to their phenolic structures.

Nickel is found in foods such as instant tea (green or black), cocoa and chocolate, crisps, wheat flour, and roasted salted cashews. Nickel is eliminated through sweat, so consumption of high concentrations of nickel can cause a cutaneous reaction. If a patient is allergic to nickel, and is suffering from vitiligo in the areas prone to sweating such as the shoulders, flanks, buttocks, and sacrum, foods containing nickel should be avoided (Han *et al*, 2005; Sharma, 2007).

Eating barbecued meats increases the production of oxygen free radicals and carcinogens in the body as well as lowers levels of antioxidants. However, most patients do not adhere to restrictions on these types of foods. Patients need to be counseled on making a modest reduction of these types of foods in their diets and maximizing antioxidant intake from vegetables and fruits. They should also cut back on fast foods and other instant foods that are high in calories and have low nutritional value. Otherwise, antioxidant supplements can also be recommended.

There are differing opinions on whether these foods are actually harmful. If a patient is to avoid all of the foods listed above, he or she could easily become more stressed and lose the benefits of a balanced diet. In our personal opinion, the various fruits or nuts mentioned above are beneficial to the patient's health and vitiligo, so we usually encourage their consumption.

Patients and doctors should pay special attention to the cutaneous reactions induced by foods. The foods listed above can cause irritation that leads to skin inflammation. It can also result in Type I anaphylactic hypersensitivity (atopic dermatitis or urticaria) and Type IV delayed hypersensitivity (allergic contact dermatitis) both of which can exacerbate vitiligo. However, these adverse events rarely occur and doctors do not need to prohibit all patients from these foods.

Furthermore, patients should rinse and wash their mouths (perioral and oral cavities) and hands after meals. Patients with celiac disease (wheat or gluten-sensitive enteropathy), in particular, those with associated dermatoses such as dermatitis herpetiformis or psoriasis, should minimize their intake of wheat because wheat or gluten can aggravate cases of vitiligo. (Humbert *et al*, 2006)

The eating habits of specific ethnic groups are also important to evaluate because certain customs can lead to skin inflammation and exacerbation of vitiligo. For example, Koreans enjoy urushiol-containing foods for gastrointestinal relief. They also eat Korean chicken or duck soup made with *Rhus* plants which can result in systemic contact dermatitis (Park *et al.* 2000). For this reason, it is necessary to perform further research studies in different regions of the world so that specific native foods that cause allergic or irritant reactions can be identified.

2.1.2 What foods are recommended?

On the whole, eating a variety of fish, meats, vegetables, and fruits is encouraged in the treatment of vitiligo. However, patients can be particular or "picky" about the foods they eat, and doctors need to take this into consideration. Meats or fish such as shark and tuna can be poisoned with dioxin, mercury, or heavy metals, which can also be problematic.

Food can serve as antioxidants. It is known that various reactive oxygen species are involved in the destruction of melanocytes in vitiligo. Many studies have shown that reactive oxygen species are increased in the epidermis of active disease. Scientists have hypothesized that elimination of these reactive oxygen species could inhibit the progression of vitiligo and studied the administration of antioxidants to patients with vitiligo. Schallreuter and colleagues (1995, 1999, 2001) reported that the combination of phototherapy and antioxidants showed a statistically significantly better response in patients compared to phototherapy alone. Recently, Dell'Anna and colleagues (2007) showed that oral supplementation with alpha-lipoic acid significantly improved the clinical effectiveness of phototherapy.

There is also further evidence for using antioxidants in the treatment of vitiligo. According to the clinical experiences of the authors, high doses of antioxidants (as part of combination treatment with other vitiligo therapies) have decreased the risk of abrupt deterioration of vitiligo. Patients with vitiligo are advised to select foods rich in antioxidants. These antioxidant-rich foods include pomegranates, grapes, oranges, lemons, grape fruits, pineapples, strawberries, kiwi, blueberries, nuts (*e.g.*, walnuts, cashew nuts), sunflower seeds, black sesame, perilla seeds, olives, black beans, tomatoes, red clover, broccoli, ginger, beets, kale, red cabbage, peppers, spinach, *Agaricus bisporus* (common/crimini mushrooms), green tea, and coffee. If the aforementioned foods are not available, patients can use commercial nutritional supplements. These include products containing genistein (black bean extract), green tea polyphenol, co-enzyme Q10, selenium, alpha-lipoic acid, omega-3 fatty acids, gamma linolenic acid, carotenoids, quercetin, vitamin C, and vitamin E, and others.

Although some specialists insist that vitamin C is harmful in vitiligo because of its skin whitening properties, we believe the advantages of vitamin C as an antioxidant outweighs the risk of hypopigmentation, and we recommend that patients to take vitamin C at a dosage of 0.5-2 grams daily.

Omega-3 fatty acids are poly-unsaturated fatty acids (PUFAs) that are known to be beneficial for psoriasis and autoimmune diseases. It may also be beneficial in vitiligo due to its anti-inflammatory, anti-oxidant, and anti-depressant effects (Simopoulos, 2002). Gamma-linolenic acid, another PUFA from evening primrose oil, is considered effective for atopic dermatitis (Kerscher & Korting, 2002). It is effective in vitiligo when vitiligo occurs with atopic dermatitis in flexural or periorbital areas, and other areas vulnerable to stimuli.

Vitamins and minerals (microelements) are also important. Some studies have demonstrated that the level of vitamin B12, folic acid, copper, and zinc in patients with vitiligo may be lower than in unaffected individuals. Microelements such as selenium, copper, and zinc are essential in the diet or as supplements. It is preferable to take vitamin B12 along with folic acid due to the considerable synergistic effects of the pairing (Jalel *et al*, 2009). It is recommended that patients obtain these nutrients from vegetables and fruits such as tomatoes, spinach, *Agaricus bisporus*, kiwi, or multivitamin supplements.

2.1.3 Food additives

Processed foods such as those found in cans or bottles, and preserved or tinned meats such as ham or sausage, contain various food additives including: dyes, color retention agents, defoaming agents, emulsifiers, flavors, fungicides, preservatives, sweeteners, thickeners, and chemicals introduced at the agricultural or animal husbandry phases, among many other possible ingredients.

While food additives are generally considered harmful in vitiligo, the medical evidence for these harmful effects is weak. In patients with atopic dermatitis, food additives like preservatives (sodium benzoate, potassium sorbate, sodium propionate), coloring agents (sodium nitrate and certain FD&C colors), or monosodium glutamate (MSG) may induce an intolerance reaction by acting on mast cells directly (Fuglsang *et al*, 1994). Consuming food additives in large amounts can also increase the risk of a stress reaction. These can have a harmful effect on vitiligo itself and accompanying skin diseases such as atopic dermatitis. Physician ought to consider the harmful effects of food additives, particularly in unstable and progressive vitiligo, although these are not so much of a concern in stable vitiligo.

2.2 Life, exercise, and stress

2.2.1 Living habits

Patients may need to change their living habits depending on their individual clinical presentation of vitiligo. For example, since severe stress can aggravate vitiligo lesions, positive thinking and reducing stress could help reduce them. Adequate rest and antioxidants are important for patients with vitiligo, particularly those with lesions in a seborrheic distribution. Patients ought to reduce smoking, a habit that siphons beneficial antioxidants from the body. It is necessary to reduce the risk of koebnerization in vitiligo through friction or trauma. For example, tight-fitting shoes or jeans, and elastic stockings should be avoided.

Identification of possible occupational trauma is important as well. Figures 2A & 2B suggest that occupational trauma such as burns or chemical irritation (*e.g.*, by discharge in an electric arc or argon welding) can exacerbate vitiligo. The patient in Figure 2C, working in a disposable mask, developed vitiligo in the perioral area where the mask was fitted. As expected, the skin lesions improved with switching to a cotton mask and excimer laser treatment for one month (Figures 2D & 2E).

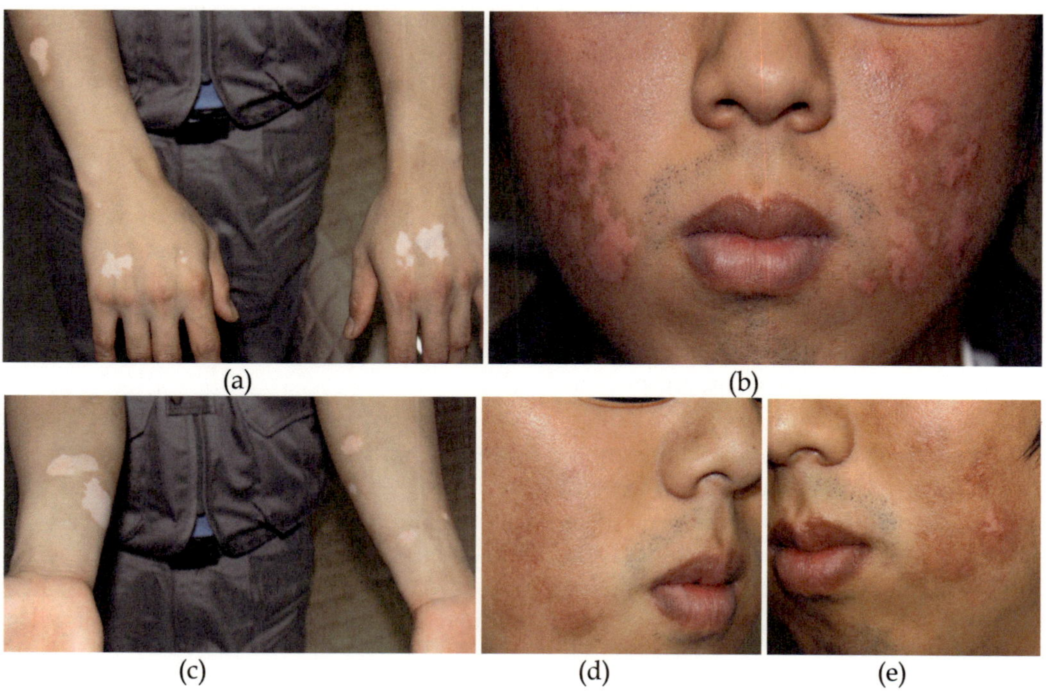

Fig. 2. (a) and (b). Occupational vitiligo induced by welding. (c) - (e). Vitiligo on areas in contact with a disposable mask, before (c) and one month after treatment (d, e)

2.2.2 UV exposure

Complementary and alternative medicine practitioners are able to take advantage of the application of photochemical reactions by treating vitiligo patients with ultraviolet rays and photosensitizers. Psoralen is the most widely used photosensitizing agent and exhibits a very strong photochemical response to ultraviolet B (UVB) as well as ultraviolet A (UVA).

Adding UVB to psoralen plus UVA (PUVA) phototherapy is an option for inducing a tremendous treatment response in vitiligo (Mofty *et al*, 2001). Similarly, exposure to sunlight (UVB and UVA), after eating or applying photosensitizing or reactive herbal medicines can cause such a strong photochemical reaction, phototoxicity, or other adverse event that can actually be used to treat vitiligo. Fragrant substances commonly cause these types of photochemical reactions. Musk or cinnamic aldehyde is widely used in cosmetics and can cause skin inflammation and worsening of vitiligo. If an inflammatory skin lesion develops, particularly on sun-exposed areas, patients should discontinue this type of product and be cautioned as to the possible photochemical reaction that occurs with exposure to sunlight.

UV therapy is a double-edged sword in the treatment of vitiligo. The pathogenesis of phototherapy with UV rays is understood in two different aspects, direct DNA damage and radical damage. First, direct DNA damage by UV rays induce the formation of cyclobutane pyrimidine dimers (CPD) as well as 6,4-photoproducts and 6,4 pyrimidine-pyrimidones that lead to skin damage. Secondly, formation of free radicals by UV rays result in damage of the skin through production of 8-oxoguanine. (Kunisada *et al*, 2007).

In particular, the shorter ultraviolet wavelengths below 305 nm more commonly bring about DNA damage and aggravate vitiligo. Since exposure to strong sunlight without sunscreen can worsen disease, patients are recommended to use sunscreens, supplement themselves with antioxidants, and avoid the use of herbal medicines, cosmetics, or herbs that can induce photochemical reactions.

2.2.3 Exercise

Repetitive movements in exercise can induce vitiligo due to trauma to or friction with certain body areas. If this is consistent with a patient's story of the appearance of certain vitiligo lesions, the patient should consider modifying or discontinuing the exercise. Common occurrences include lesions of the dorsal shin in soccer, inner thigh and groin for horseback riders, protuberant areas in contact with protective headgear, and pressure points on the hands and palms when gripping golf clubs.

2.3 Other dermatoses and vitiligo: Atopic dermatitis and allergic contact dermatitis

Patients with vitiligo can exhibit sensitivity or form an allergic response to a variety of chemicals and products that can lead to aggravation of vitiligo.

For example, some patients have shown marked improvement of vitiligo lesions in the forehead and scalp region after changing their paraphenylene diamine (PPDA)-based hair dyes to dyes that did not contain the ingredient and therefore were not allergic or sensitive to.

Considering reports of the deterioration of vitiligo after imiquimod treatment, it is desirable to avoid imiquimod if possible.

Patients who are allergic to nickel should avoid contact with the metal as it is contained in many accessories and jewelry. If patients insist on continuing to wear such accessories, they can switch to those that are nickel-free (*e.g.*, titanium).

Cosmetics and oral hygiene products can cause problems in vitiligo. There are many cases in which patients improve after using paraben- or fragrance-free products (personal communication with Prof. Ai-Young Lee, Dong-kuk University, Ilsan, Korea, and authors' experience). Patients and doctors need to decide whether to continue the use of these products considering the distribution of vitiligo lesions, the areas to which the products are applied, and based on the results of patch testing of specific products.

The patient in Figure 3A developed vitiligo only in the lip and perioral region. Patch testing was positive for thimerosal. She showed much improvement in skin lesions after discontinuing the use of mouthwashes and toothpastes containing thimerosal and using thimerosal-free products.

Enough rest and appropriate treatment can help vitiligo in the "T-zone" areas where seborrheic dermatitis commonly occurs. If a lesion appears in areas which have a predilection for atopic dermatitis, doctors should pay special attention to treatment of the skin lesion. Adjunctive use of ketotifen and gamma-linolenic acid is useful. For the patient in Figure 3B, phototherapy as well as treatment for atopic dermatitis and diaper dermatitis would be necessary.

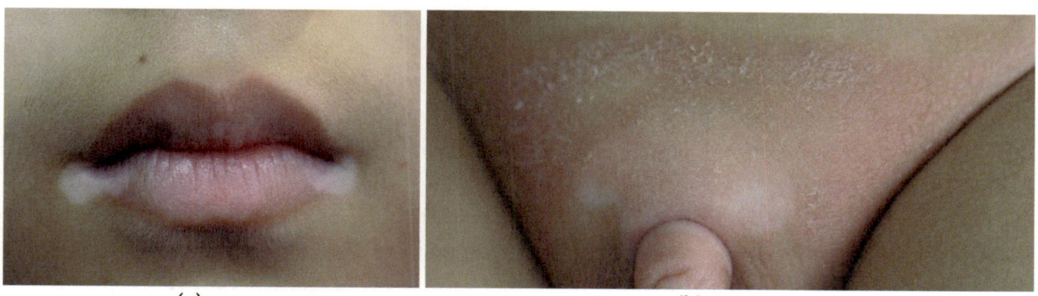

(a) (b)

Fig. 3. A. Vitiligo on angles of mouth. B. Vitiligo associated with atopic dermatitis and diaper dermatitis.

2.4 Aesthetic treatment and vitiligo

Many patients suffering from vitiligo want purely aesthetic treatment, which can be harmful. IPL (intense pulsed light) can induce vitiligo (Shin *et al*, 2010). Authors have experienced cases of vitiligo aggravated after monopolar and bipolar radiofrequency treatments (Tenor, Alma) for rejuvenation, as well as low fluence Q-switched Nd-YAG laser for the treatment of melasma. Since keratinocytes in vitiligo are highly sensitive to stimuli (Lee *et al*, 2005), aesthetic treatment should be reserved for stable vitiligo at periods when a patient is less stressed, and at a relatively shallow depth of penetration, *i.e.*, by narrowing the interval and width of pulse of IPL and lowering the fluence of Nd: YAG laser. Doctors must be discreet in utilizing laser treatments and consider the activity and severity of vitiligo of the patients who inquire about elective cosmetic treatments.

3. Complementary and alternative medicine (CAM) for vitiligo

3.1 Traditional Chinese medicine (TCM)

The history of TCM dates back thousands of years. The variety and usage of these medicines is almost identical throughout Korea, China, and Japan thanks to long-term cultural exchange among nations (Bark *et al*, 2010).

According to TCM, wind (climate), wetness (humidity), and coldness (temperature) invade the skin and inhibit the cycle of energy and blood, and can cause discordances among them. The blockage of energy and blood paves the way for diseases, which has a cumulative effect with various internal and external factors (*e.g.*, stress, coldness). The discordance of energy and blood inhibits nutrient delivery to the skin, and allows bad spirits to invade, resulting in vitiligo. For this reason, TCM doctors insist that the recovery of circulation of energy and blood can cure vitiligo. TCM places an emphasis on the effects of *decoctions* of herbs rather than that of each herb. Some oriental herbs have different names depending on the parts utilized (*e.g.*, stalk or root) as well as preparation (*e.g.*, peeled or unpeeled, steamed or dried). Furthermore, recent studies show that there are differences in the end product which are dependent on processing methods and parts utilized. For ginseng (*Panax)*, one of the most studied plants, the main ingredient ginsenoside is altered by different processing methods such as drying and steam-drying which alter them from the raw product. Each ginsenoside has a different medical mechanism of action and the effect of each has been identified (Choi, 2008; Kim *et al*, 2007).

Among the decoctions of herbs which TCM primarily uses, the most effective medicines have been shown to be the xiaobailing decoction, Chang-yee powder, and three-yellow powder. These medicines include various medicinal plants such as *Xanthium strumarium*, *Sophora flavescens*, *Atractylodes japonica*, and *Arisaema amurense*. The TCM medicines known to be effective in vitiligo are listed in Table 1.

According to Bark *et al* (2010), a quarter of 64 TCM plants have been shown to have phototoxic properties. They show strong fluorescence in phototoxicity tests and are positive in photohemolysis and *Candida albicans* tests. In a mouse experiment with 5 TCM plants, the UVA plus TCM group showed phototoxic reactions such as skin swelling, sunburn cell formation, depletion of Langerhans cells, and suppression of local contact hypersensitivity to dinitrofluorobenzene (DNFB).

Additionally, a study of 160 TCM medicines revealed the number of phototoxic drugs at a similar ratio to the previous study (Bark *et al*, in preparation). Because a number of herbal medicines have different absorbance and fluorescence patterns than psoralen, they can be considered as alternative photosensitizing agents for photochemotherapy. The phototoxic properties of *Xanthium strumarium* and *Psoralea corylifolia* have been shown to be stronger than those of psoralen (authors' unpublished data). Table 1 includes some of the medicines that the authors have examined and determined to be phototoxic.

The effectiveness of TCM is considerably lower than that of modern medicine. TCM may include harmful or ineffective components because it uses a decoction of components. Therefore, safety is our priority in TCM. Many people have consumed TCM without any safety monitoring, believing it to be a secret method passed from generation-to-generation for thousands of years. This ideology can be harmful. The use of *Aristolochia fangchi* resulted in European patients developing renal failure and kidney cancer when taken as an obesity treatment. (Arlt *et al*, 2002; Cosyns *et al*, 1994; Vanherweghem *et al*, 1993). It is necessary to further study the efficacy and safety of TCM.

Arsenic or mercury used in TCM can be effective for vitiligo, but these are dangerous materials. Even now, many Koreans develop arsenic keratosis after receiving TCM therapy previously (Figure 4). Furthermore, arsenic can also be absorbed though the skin (Lowney *et al*, 2005). The bigger issue is that the Korean Food & Drug Administration approved arsenic and mercury for TCM therapy (2007).

Scientific Name	Common name or Ayurvedic name	Proposed mechanism of action
Angelica sinensis		phototoxic
Arisaema amurense		antioxidant
Astragalus membranaceus		
Atractylodes japonica		phototoxic
Carthamus tinctorius	safflower	antioxidant
Cassia occidentalis	kasaundi, stinking weed	melanoblast differentiation and migration
Cnidium officinale	chuanxiong rhizome	phototoxic
Codonopsis pilosula	Tangshen	
Cuscuta chinensis/japonica	dodder seed	antioxidant
Eclipta prostrata	bhangrah	antioxidant
Gentiana scabra		anti-inflammatory
Liquidambar formosana	sweetgum fruit	promotes circulation
Lycium chinense	wolfberry fruit	nutrient, antioxidant
Paeonia lactiflora	white peony root	
Paeonia lactiflora	red peony root	
Picrorhiza kurroa	Katuki, kutki	phototoxic
Pleuropterus multiflorus		promotes circulation, antioxidant
Polygala tenuifolia		phototoxic
Prunella vulgaris	prunella spike	immunomodulatory effects
Prunus persica	peach kernel	
Rehmania glutinosa	Chinese foxglove	nutrient, antioxidant
Salvia miltiorrhiza	red sage	antioxidant, anti-inflammatory, promotes circulation
scorpion		toxin?
Sesamum indicum	black sesame	antioxidant
Sophora flavescens		
Spatholobus suberectus	climbing stem of *S. suberectus*	promotes circulation
Spirodela polyrhiza		
Tribulus terrestris	gokshura, sarrata	phototoxic
Xanthium strumarium		phototoxic

Table 1. Complementary and Alternative Medicines Utilized in Vitiligo

Koreans consider and take herbal medicine as health food. Dozens of cases of vitiligo exacerbations were observed in those taking high dose supplements of ginseng products like raw ginseng, red ginseng, white ginseng, and products from the *Acanthopanax species* (*A. sessiliflorum, A. gracilistylus, A. senticosus*), and *Phellinus linteusau* (mushroom) for over one month. Therefore, patients and doctors must keep in mind that these medicines can affect immune status and aggravate vitiligo. Consuming small amounts of ginseng products or applying them to the skin can improve vitiligo. Nevertheless, it is more beneficial not to use these in terms of potential risks involved.

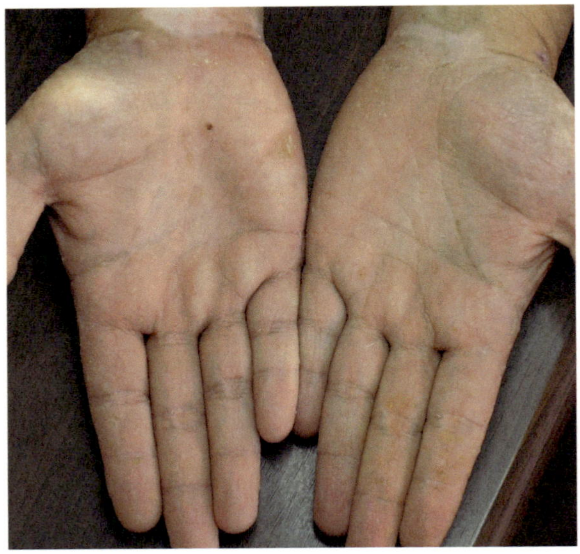

Fig. 4. Arsenic keratoses in vitiligo patient

3.2 Traditional Indian medicine

Traditional Indian medicine has thousands of years of history. Its branches include Ayurveda, Yoga & Naturopathy, Unani, and Siddha medicine. Due to a long history of active trading between China and India through the Silk Road (via Central Asia, trans-Himalayan, or sea-route), there are similarities in the medicinal plants utilized and their indications. *Cassia occidentalis, Eclipta prostrata, Curcuma longa, Picrorrhiza kurroa, Psoralea corylifolia*, and *Tribulus terrestris* are commonly used in both Ayurvedic medicine and TCM (Dharmananda, 2011).

However, there are fundamental differences between Ayurveda and TCM. Despite having common drugs, Ayurvedic medicine and TCM use them for different applications. Ayurvedic medicine primarily uses mineral-based and herbal drugs that act as photosensitizers and blood purifiers (Srivastava, 2011).

Photosensitizing agents include *Psoralea corylifolia, Semicarpus anacardium* (marking nut), and *Ficus hispida*. They are administrated locally as well as systematically in conjunction with sun exposure. Sun exposure is advised three hours after drug administration. Blood purifiers include *Curcuma longa, Eclipta alba, Tinospora cardifolia, Hemidascus indicus, Acasia catachu*, and *Acaranthus aspara* (Srivastava, 2011).

Traditional Siddha medicine uses *Aristolochia indica, Tribulus terrestris*, and *Thespesia populnea* (Soni *et al*, 2010). Among these, *Aristolochia indica* root contains aristolochic acid, so it can cause a renal failure or cancer. (Arlt *et al*, 2002; Cosyns *et al*, 1994; Vanherweghem *et al*, 1993). Both the hepatotoxicity of *Psoralea corylifolia* (Teschke & Bahre, 2009, Cheung *et al*, 2009), and its phototoxicity (Bark *et al*, 2010) are mentioned due to its possible applications in vitiligo. Ayurvedic medicine as well as TCM acknowledge the risks of the use of arsenic and mercury (Saper *et al*, 2004).

Ayurvedic doctors recommend that patients avoid tea, coffee, alcoholic beverages, oranges, sweet lime, sea food, excessive salt, and sour or fermented food products. However, these foods have not been observed to cause any deterioration in vitiligo patients, and in fact, tea, red wine, orange, or fermented foods seem to be rather helpful for vitiligo. More studies should be performed to identify the efficacy of these foods.

3.3 Homeopathic treatment

Homeopathy is a form of alternative medicine that originated in 18th century Germany. Many countries have adapted and transformed these practices in accordance to their cultures. India is particularly well known for its wide application of various homeopathic treatments that claim a high "cure" rates, but there is a lack of medical evidence substantiating this. Poisonous materials such as arsenic sulph falvus, arsenic album (arsenic trioxide), baryta muriaticum (barium chloride) and baryta carbonicum (barium Carbonate), are often employed by practitioners in highly diluted preparations. The collective weight of scientific evidence has found homeopathy to be no more effective than placebo.

3.4 Folk remedies in Korea

There are various Korean folk remedies for vitiligo. Apart from TCM, folk remedies include the root of *Rumex crispus* or leaves of the common fig tree (*Ficus carica*) which contain strong phototoxic agents (mainly furocoumarine). These phototoxic agents are less effective than modern medicine (*i.e.*, psoralen) because these preparations are affected by many variables, such as active ingredient concentration, treatment frequency, and application or administration methods.

Foreign body reactions using various irritants that add pigment to the skin (*i.e.*, tattooing) are often harmful and have no benefits. Bee venom is regarded as ineffective and dangerous because it induces systemic inflammation. However, *purified* honey bee venom (apitoxin) may be effective in vitiligo (Jeon *et al*, 2007).

Rhododendron schlippenbachii and *Lespedeza bicolor* show significant improvement in vitiligo lesions when applied topically or combined with phototherapy. Though the mechanism of action has not been clearly elucidated, it is presumably related to the activation of melanocytes and the effect of antioxidants or toxins (*e.g.*, alkaloid, rhodoxin, andromedotoxin) (HY Kang, JK Yang, TH Kim, in preparation).

3.5 Suggested mechanisms of action of complementary and alternative treatments

Table 1 lists CAM therapeutics used for treatment of vitiligo. It is unclear by which mechanisms these medicines use in vitiligo. The authors do not support the motion of energy theorem suggested in TCM or Ayurvedic medicine. In modern medicine and dermatology, phototoxic reactions, melanocyte proliferation, promoting anti-inflammatory activity, and trigger reduction (*e.g.*, stress, environmental factors) are thought to be involved in vitiligo management.

Ammi visnaga (khellin), *Angelica sinensis, Atractylodes japonica, Cnidium officinale, Ficus carca, Ficus hispida, Hypericium sp., Picrorhiza kurroa, Polygala tenuifolia, Psoralea corylifolia, Rumex crispus, Semicarpus anacardium, Tribulus terrestris,* and *Xanthium strumarium* have phototoxic properties. Like psoralen, they can be combined with relevant ultraviolet rays or sunlight (Bark *et al*, 2010; Bark *et al*, in preparation; Srivastava, 2011).

Bee venom, *Angelicae dahuricae, Astragalus membranaceus, Cassia occidentalis, Cuscuta chinensis, Flos Carthami, Psoralea corylifolia, Lespedeza bicolor, Ligustrum lucidum, Malytea scurfpea,*

Rhododendron schlippenbachii, *Salvia miltiorrhiza*, and *Tribulus terrestris* are known to induce melanocyte proliferation, melanogenesis, and migration of melanocytes.
There has been reports of the antioxidant effects of black sesame, *Arisaema amurense*, *Carthamus tinctorius*, *Cuscuta chinensis/japonica*, *Eclipta prostrata*, *Lycium chinense*, *Pleuropterus multiflorus*, *Psoralea corylifolia*, *Rehmania glutinosa*, and *Salvia miltiorrhiza*, among others. More studies should be performed to further evaluate the antioxidant effects of these medicines.

3.6 Commercial therapeutics for vitiligo

There are many products on the market which are targeted to patients with vitiligo. However, the efficacy and safety of these products are questionable and the authors do not particularly recommend the use of any of these products.
Vitiligo Herb™ and **Anti-Vitiligo™** contain coconut oil, *Psoralea corylifolia*, black cumin, and barberry root. *Psoralea coryli* has strongly phototoxic properties. Barbery root (*Berberis vulgaris*) containing isoquinoline alkaloid (berberine) has antioxidant and anti-inflammatory effects, and inhibits the COX-2 enzyme. Other ingredients included in these products are purported to be antioxidants or nutrients. These products *could* potentiate the effects of phototherapy or sun exposure. Unless patients understand the concerns of using photosensitizers with phototherapy and heliotherapy, treatment using these products can be dangerous.
Low levels of catalase in the epidermis of patients who have vitiligo increase hydrogen peroxide (H_2O_2) levels, which inhibits 6-BH4 metabolism and melanogenesis. Shallreuter and colleagues (1995, 1999, 2001) suggest that antioxidants are effective for vitiligo. They reported that topical application of **pseudocatalase** and calcium in combination with UVB resulted in complete repigmentation of the face and back of the hands in 90% of a cohort of patients. However, Patel *et al* (2002) used a pseudocatalase and calcium combined with narrowband UVB (NB-UVB), and found no clear evidence of efficacy. It is unclear the differences which come from different manufacturing methods. There is controversy as to whether the effects of *Cucumis melo* extracts are similar to pseudocatalase. *Cucumis melo* extracts have shown to have vitiligo-relevant superoxide-dismutase and catalase-like activities when used with selective UVB therapy (Kostović *et al*, 2007). However, it was ineffective in other studies (Schallreuter & Rokos, 2005; Yuksel *et al*, 2009).
"Callumae" is a product which contains *Picrorhiza kurroa*, khellin, L-phenylalanine, gingko biloba, alpha lipoic acid, cyanocobalamin, pyridoxine and folic acid. Among these, *Picrorhiza kurroa* and khellin have psoralen-like phototoxic properties while L-phenylalanine has been shown to be effective for vitiligo combined with UVA phototherapy. Gingko biloba and alpha lipoic acid are known to be a natural source of antioxidants. Cyanocobalamin, pyridoxine, and folic acid are vitamins which have shown some usefulness in vitiligo. A combination of phototherapy plus these products may produce greater efficacy.
Phenylalanine, an essential amino acid, is precursor for tyrosine, the monoamine signaling molecules dopamine, norepinephrine, epinephrine, and the skin pigment melanin. There is moderate evidence that L-phenylalanine has efficacy as an adjunct to phototherapy. L-phenylalanine plus UVA (50-100 mg/kg + UVA twice weekly 30-45 min after ingestion) provided better results than L-phenylalanine alone (Siddiqui *et al*, 1994). However, some adverse events have been attributed to L-phenylalanine (Rosenbach *et al*, 1993).
"Vitilax" is a mixture of many ingredients known to be effective for vitiligo (Table 1). Its ingredients include *Psoralea corylifolia*, *Astragalus membranaceus*, Chinese peony root, *Cnidium* fruit, Chinese *Salvia* root and rhizome, *Tribulus fruit*, Chinese dodder seed, Fo-Ti root (polygonum), turmeric root (*Curcuma longa*), atractylodes rhizome, dong quai root

(*Angelica sinensis*), safflower (*Carthamus tinctorius*), fragrant *Angelica* root, and cassia twig (*Cassia occidentalis*).

Khellin is extracted from the seeds of the plant *Ammi visnaga*. Since 1982, khellin has been proposed as an oral photochemotherapy treatment for vitiligo (Abdel-Fattah *et al.* 1982). Fiver percent khellin in water/oil is applied to a vitiliginous lesion and an hour later, UVA (KUVA) was administered. The control group was treated with conventional systemic PUVA with oral psoralen (0.4 mg/kg). The study showed that both KUVA and PUVA treatment had similar efficacy, but since KUVA is given locally, there may be less risk involved.

Polypodium leucotomos extract (FernBlock®) is a potent antioxidant. Since oxidative stress has been implicated in the vitiligo, it has been used in vitiligo. It was shown to be effective as monotherapy or in combination with NB-UVB (Middelkamp-Hup *et al*, 2007).

"Melagenina I and II" (placental extract) has been used topically primarily in combination with sun exposure to repigment vitiligo lesions. Its efficacy is questionable, but in recent study, the efficacy of NB-UVB plus topical placental extract caused a modest but statistically insignificant improvement in vitiligo than NB-UVB alone (Majid, 2010).

Ginkgo biloba has antioxidant and immunomodulatory properties. *Ginkgo biloba* extracts given orally can prevent the active progression of vitiligo and induce repigmentation (Parsad *et al*, 2003; Szczurko *et al*, 2011). Considering the mechanism of action of *Ginko biloba*, combination with phototherapy would theoretically be more effective than *Ginko biloba* alone.

Novitil® contains lipoproteins, polypeptides, *Aloe barbadensis*, carboxymethylcellulose, camphor, menthol and oligoelements. Only *aloe barbadensis* may have anti-inflammatory activity in vitiligo, but other ingredients listed do not have proven anti-vitiligo effects.

3.7 Other treatments

Serrano *et al* (2009) reported that repeated photodynamic therapy (PDT) with low concentrations of aminolevulinic acid (ALA, 1-2%) is helpful in the vitiligo. We have had similar experiences in patients with alopecia totalis. We treated patients with a very low concentration of ALA (0.5%), and asked them to wait 2 hours before exposing themselves to window glass-filtered sunlight for 30 minutes once every two weeks. If similar treatment is repeated in vitiligo, it may work. This may be due to the protoporphyrin IX produced by ALA that strongly absorbs UVA.

Aghaei and Ardekani (2008) reported that diphenylcyclopropenone (DPCP) showed some efficacy in the treatment of vitiligo. DPCP is thought to act as a local irritant when applied topically. However, based on our clinical experience, this agent seems to be quite dangerous and unreliable. There are reports of vitiligo occurring after treatment with DPCP for alopecia areata (Hatzis *et al*, 1988; Pires *et al*, 2010). The authors have also experienced some cases of deterioration of vitiligo in patients treated with DPCP for their alopecia totalis or molluscum contagiosum.

4. Camouflage of vitiligo

4.1 Introduction

The majority of patients who suffer from vitiligo want to conceal their exposed vitiligo lesions because of psychosocial reasons. Patients conceal lesions on the face, head and neck, arms, legs, and hands with clothing or other methods. Concealment is a useful way to improve social functioning and patient quality of life (Tanioka *et al*, 2010). Camouflage can take the form of: micropigmentation which lasts for months to years (tattoos and semi-permanent tattoos/permanent makeup), dihydroxyacetone and selected fruit juices that last for several days, and dyes or makeup concealers which last for 1- 2 days.

4.2 Long-acting camouflage; Micropigmentation

Micropigmentation is a method in which pigments are injected directly into dermis and last for months to years at a time. This can be in the form of tattooing or semi-permanent tattoos (permanent makeup) depending on the features of pigments utilized.

Tattoos have been used widely throughout the world for thousands of years, as part of cultural and ethnic activities to recreational purposes. In vitiligo, the pigments that have been used in vitiligo include mercury (red), lead (yellow, green, white), cadmium (red, orange, yellow), nickel (black), zinc (yellow, white), titanium (white), iron (brown, red, black), barium (white), and carbon (black). Organic chemicals, including azo-chemicals (orange, brown, yellow, green, violet) and naptha-derived chemicals have been used. Elements such as antimony, arsenic, beryllium, calcium, lithium, selenium, and sulfur are also employed.

Tattoo ink manufacturers typically make either blends of heavy metal pigments or lightening agents (such as lead or titanium). This method has the advantage of long-lasting effects. This is useful particularly for lesions on the scalp, eyebrows, and lips, which are naturally pigmented. However, it is difficult to adjust or homogenize tone of skin color, and the results are often unsatisfactory.

Some skillful tattooists provide cosmetically good results to patients. Singh & Karki (2010) obtained cosmetically acceptable results in tattooing Indian patients who had localized, stable vitiligo on their lips. Permanent makeup is similar to conventional (temporary) makeup (*e.g.*, concealer) and is preferred by patients who want to look natural (De Cuyper, 2008). For most Koreans, pigment lasts for approximately 2-4 years, according to the authors' experience with hundreds of such cases. However, as the semi-permanent makeup fades, it leaves a reddish tint in treated areas.

Permanent makeup uses digitalized tattoo machines and need re-touching when colors begin to fade after treatment (around one month).

The primary pigments may be excreted slowly by trans-epidermal elimination. It can be predicted that the pigments deposited at the dermal papilla are much more likely to disappear gradually similarly to the mechanism by which amyloid deposition in the dermal papillae emits outward through transepidermal elimination in primary localized cutaneous amyloidosis (Kibbi *et al*, 1992). The longevity of individual pigments seems to be dependent upon composition. When red residue remains after a tattoo fades, it is after the disappearance of plant-derived organic dyes.

Permanent makeup has the advantage of lasting for a long time. Eyebrows or lips can be concealed naturally with permanent makeup. Since it is difficult to homogenize or adjust the varying skin tones for each individual, therapists make a lighter shade of color than they desire with permanent makeup and then add conventional makeup with concealer. Pigments used for diluting colors are often left in the skin for a long time. In the case of titanium dioxide, patients can experience paradoxical darkening, which is cosmetically undesirable, although dermatologists have successfully treated this with the Q-switch laser (Kirby *et al*, 2010).

The common problem with **micropigmentation** is dissatisfaction with shape and tone. It is difficult for even the most experienced tattooists to make pigments with accurate tone, depths, and symmetry, particularly for the eyebrows and lips. The deeply injected pigment can develop an unnatural look due to the Tyndall effect (scattering of light). Furthermore, due to trauma in micropigmentation procedures, koebnerization leading to vitiligo can occur. Furthermore, adverse events are a possibility with these procedures, and include infection, allergic reactions, tattoo granulomas, keloid formation, and magnetic resonance imaging (MRI) complications. Magnetic responsive dyes in tattoo can cause cutaneous reactions when patients undergo MRI testing. (De Cuyper, 2008; FDA, 2011; Kirby 2010).

4.3 Intermediate-acting camouflage

Dihydroxyacetone (DHA) is an ingredient in self-tanning products. This dyeing method camouflages lesions of vitiligo temporarily because of browning by the Maillard reaction (Fusaro & Rice, 2005). DHA can mask lesions of vitiligo relatively well and lasts for 3-6 days. (Rajatanavin *et al*, 2008; Suga *et al*, 2002).

According to our experience, many patients combine DHA with conventional makeup. Korean patients with vitiligo effectively conceal lesions using DHA concentrations of 5-15%. Since DHA can make lesions slightly reddish brown, it is not well-suited for patients with yellow skin tones.

DHA is not very effective in damaged or inflamed stratum corneum. It may also interfere with the effects of phototherapy by inhibiting ultraviolet rays (Fusaro & Rice, 2005). Patients need to practice application techniques for the most natural-appearing camouflage because final coloring appears several hours after application.

Applying a dye from premature walnut shells is a natural pigmentation aid for vitiligo. Premature walnut shells are frozen and made into a solution. This can further be diluted to match skin color, in particular for patients with yellow undertones. However, this method can cause an allergic contact dermatitis (due to the walnut shell), and due to the instability of the dye solution, it becomes less effective after a day.

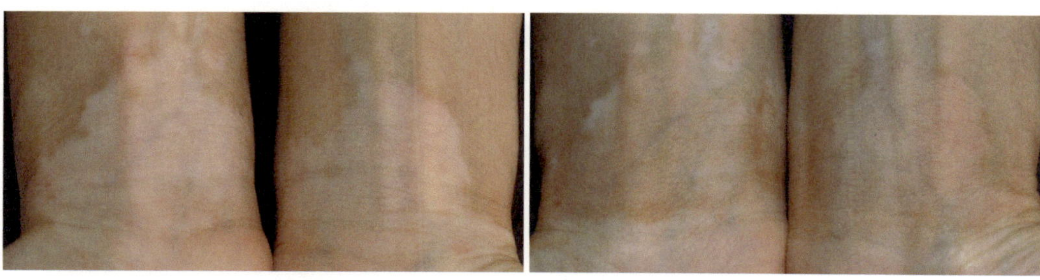

Fig. 5. Concealing with 7.5% dihydroxyacetone (left), and walnut shell extract (right). A. Before concealing. B. After concealing.

Figure 5 compares the effects of DHA solution versus that of walnut shell. The patient preferred DHA (Figure 1B, left) due to its more natural and longer-lasting effects. However, some patients do prefer the walnut shell-derived dye.

Henna (made from mehndi leaves) is sometimes recommended for vitiligo, however, the stain is generally more red than naturally occurring skin tones. Henna with a brown or black color contains added paraphenylene diamine which can often cause an allergic contact dermatitis and aggravate vitiligo.

4.4 Short-acting camouflage

Dyes such as potassium permanganate, indigo carmine, and bismarck brown can be used to camouflage vitiligo. These dyes provide an immediate, natural, amber-like shade with single or repeated applications, and can be easily removed by washing (Sarveswari, 2010).

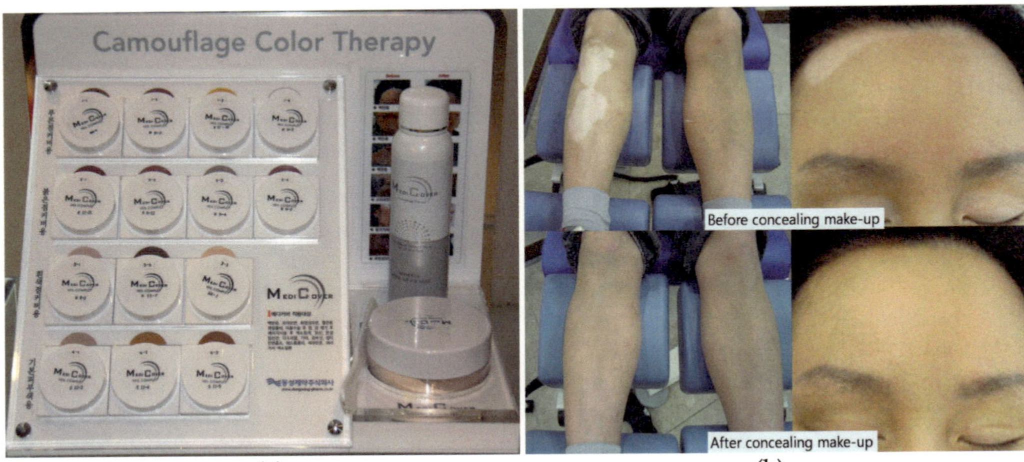

(a) (b)

Fig. 6. (a). Concealer cosmetic set for vitiligo patients. (b). Patient before and after makeup. Courtesy of Dong-Sung Pharmaceutical, Co., Seoul, Korea.

Special makeup products are also helpful. Cosmetics are limited by their easy removability (can be washed away by sweat) and they can be messy (get on clothing), however tend to give vitiligo lesions the most natural skin color. Many patients prefer makeup, which can achieve cosmetically acceptable results in an investment of 20 minutes a day. Special makeup is acceptable, but it is more effective when combined with DHA or walnut solution. Figure 6 shows a patient before and after makeup. To maintain the stability of makeup where it is applied, non-glossy hair spray (Korean) or Cavilon 3M™ spray (Tanioka & Miyachi, 2008) can be used after application of makeup. Some KAV patients use spray-on stockings on a DHA-primed leg lesion and results are often satisfactory. However, it is difficult for beginners to produce satisfactory results using various makeup products. The methods using DHA, walnut shell, and special makeup products all require hours of patient teaching and practice. Tanioka and Miyachi (2009) also emphasized the importance of lessons in camouflage techniques.

In terms of products for camouflage, a number of brands are available, including Dermablend™, Covermark™, Derma Color™, Dermage™, Elizabeth Arden Concealing Cream™, and Medi-Cover™. These are concealer-type cosmetics that are not easily washed away by sweat and come in a variety of skin colors.

Drula Pigment Cream™, Viti-color™, DY-O-Derm Vitiligo™, Chromelin Complexion Blender™, Mela-Pen™, Vitiligo Cover™ are also products for camouflage containing dihydroxyacetone (DHA). Drula Pigment Cream™ and Viti-color™ contains erythrulose, which has long-lasting effects. Vitiligo Cover™ contains both DHA and walnut shell.

5. Conclusion

Patients and doctors can safely combine modern medicines with reliable CAM all while encouraging healthy lifestyles in order to prevent vitiligo exacerbation. CAM is less effective for vitiligo compared to modern medicine although it has shown some merit in making use of the phototoxic, anti-congestion, anti-oxidant, anti-stress, and immune modulation properties of specific herbs and herbal combinations. Various natural foods and products can be another option for the treatment of vitiligo. Additionally, patients and doctors must consider the often unexpected side effects of these products due to their unregulated ingredients. On the whole, topical treatment with CAM is relatively safe and effective. Camouflage is an efficient method for vitiligo in terms of cost-benefit ratio and improving quality of life. Various CAM modalities including TCM, health foods, good living habits, and camouflage combined with Western medicine, in the form of oral or topical medications, phototherapy, or excimer laser, can help these patients live happier lives with decreased disease burden.

6. References

Abdel-Fattah, A.; Aboul-Enein, MN.; Wassel, GM. & El-Menshawi, BS. (1982). An approach to the treatment of vitiligo by khellin. *Dermatologica*. Vol.165, No.2, (August 1982), pp 136-140.

Aghaei, S. & Ardekani, GS. (2008). Topical immunotherapy with diphenylcyclopropenone in vitiligo: a preliminary experience. *Indian J Dermatol Venereol Leprol*. Vol.74, No.6, (November 2008), pp628-631.

Alikhan, A.; Felsten, LM.; Daly, M. & Petronic-Rosic, V. (2011). Vitiligo: A comprehensive overview Part I. Introduction, epidemiology, quality of life, diagnosis, differential diagnosis, associations, histopathology, etiology, and work-up. *J Am Acad Dermatol*. Vol.65, No.3, (September 2011), pp473-491.

Arlt, VM.; Stiborova, M. & Schmeiser, HH. Aristolochic acid as a probable human cancer hazard in herbal remedies: a review. *Mutagenesis*. Vol.14, No.4, (July 2002), pp265-277.

Bark, KM.; Heo, EP.; Han KD.; Kim, MB.; Lee, ST.; Gil, EM. & Kim, TH. (2010). Evaluation of the phototoxic potential of plants used in oriental medicine. *J Ethnopharmacol*. Vol.127, No.1, (January 2010), pp11-18.

Cheung, WI.; Tse, ML.; Ngan, T.; Lin, J.; Lee, WK.; Poon, WT.; Mak, TW.; Leung, VK. & Chau, TN. (2009). Liver injury associated with the use of Fructus Psoraleae (Bol-gol-zhee or Bu-gu-zhi) and its related proprietary medicine. *Clin Toxicol (Phila)*. Vol.47, No.7, (August 2009), pp683-685.

Choi, KT. (2008). Botanical characteristics, pharmacological effects and medicinal components of Korean Panax ginseng C A Meyer. *Acta pharmacol Sin*. Vol.29, No.9, (September 2008), pp1109-1118.

Cosyns, JP.; Jadoul, M.; Squifflet JP.; De Plaen, JF.; Ferluga, D. & van Ypersele de Strihou, C. (1994). Chinese herbs nephropathy: a clue to Balkan endemic nephropathy? *Kidney Int*. Vol.46, No.6, (June 1994), pp1680-1688.

Dharmananda, S. (August, 2011). Ayurvedic Herbal Medicine and its Relation to Chinese Herbal Medicine, 22/08/2011, Available from http://www.itmonline.org/arts/ayurherb.htm

De Cuyper, C. (2008). Permanent makeup: indications and complications. *Clin Dermatol*. Vol.26, No.1, (January 2008), pp30-34.

Dell'Anna, ML.; Mastrofrancesco, A.; Sala, R. *et al.* (2007). Antioxidants and narrow band-UVB in the treatment of vitiligo: a double-blind placebo controlled trial. *Clin Exp Dermatol*. Vo.32, No.6, (November 2007), pp631-636.

FDA. (August 2011). Tattoos & Permanent Makeup. In: *Cosmetics*, 22,08,2011, Available from http://www.fda.gov/Cosmetics/ProductandIngredientSafety /ProductInformation/ucm108530.htm

Felsten, LM.; Alikhan, A. & Petronic-Rosic, V. (2011). Vitiligo: A comprehensive overview Part II: Treatment options and approach to treatment. *J Am Acad Dermatol*. Vol.65, No.3, (September 2011), pp493-514.

Fusaro, RM. & Rice, EG. (2005). The maillard reaction for sunlight protection. *Ann N Y Acad Sci*. Vol.1043, (June 2005), 174-183.

Fuglsang, G.; Madsen, G.; Halken, S.; Jørgensen, S.; Ostergaard, PA. & Osterballe, O. (1994). Adverse reactions to food additives in children with atopic symptoms. *Allergy*. vol.49, No.1, (January 1994), pp31-37.

Han, HJ.; Lee, BH.; Park, CW.; Lee, CH. & Kang, YS. (2005). A study of Nickel Content in Korean Foods. *Korean J Dermatol*. Vol.43, No.5, (May 2005), pp593-598.

Hatzis, J.; Gourgiotou, K.; Tosca, A.; Varelzidis, A. & Stratigos, J. (1988). Vitiligo as a reaction to topical treatment with diphencyprone. *Dermatologica*. Vol.177, No.3, (September 1988), pp146-148.

Humbert, P.; Pelletier, F.; Dreno, B.; Puzenat, E. & Aubin, F. (2006). Gluten intolerance and skin diseases. *Eur J Dermatol*. Vol.16, No.1, (January 2006), pp4-11.

Jalel, A.; Soumaya, GS. & Hamdaoui, MH. (2009). Vitiligo treatment with vitamins, minerals and polyphenol supplementation. *Indian J Dermatol*. Vol.54, No.4, (October 2009), pp357-360.

Jeon, S.; Kim, NH.; Koo, BS.; Lee, HJ. & Lee, AY. (2007). Bee venom stimulates human melanocyte proliferation, melanogenesis, dendricity and migration. *Exp Mol Med*. Vol.39, No.5, (October 2007), pp603-613.

Kerscher, MJ. & Korting, HC. (1992). Treatment of atopic eczema with evening primrose oil: rationale and clinical results. *Clin Investig*. Vol.70, No.2, (February 1992), pp167-171.

Kibbi, AG.; Rubeiz, NG.; Zaynoun, ST. & Kurban, AK. (1992). Primary localized cutaneous amyloidosis. *Int J Dermatol*. Vol.32, No.2, (February 1992), pp95-98.

Kim, SN.; Ha, YW.; Shin, H. *et al*. (2007). Simultaneous quantification of 14 ginsenosides in Panax ginseng C.A. Meyer (Korean red ginseng) by HPLC-ELSD and its application to quality control. *J Pharm Biomed Anal*. Vol.45, No.1, (September 2007), pp164-170.

Kirby, W.; Kaur, RR. & Desai, A. (2010). Paradoxical darkening and removal of pink tattoo ink. J Cosmet Dermatol. Vol.9, No.2, (June 2010), pp149-151.

Korean Food & Drug Administration. (2007). *Instruction guide for safe use of Korean traditional medicine - mercuric sulfide, orpiment (arsenic)*. (in Korean. Title translated by authors). Government Publications Registration Number (Korea) 11-1470000-001464-14, Seoul, Korea

Kostović, K.; Pastar, Z.; Pasić, A. & Ceović, R. (2007). Treatment of vitiligo with narrow-band UVB and topical gel containing catalase and superoxide dismutase. Acta Dermatovenerol Croat. Vol.15, No.1, (January 2007), pp10-14.

Kunisada, M.; Kumimoto, H.; Ishizaki, K.; Sakumi, K.; Nakabeppu, Y. & Nishigori, C. (2007). Narrow-band UVB induces more carcinogenic skin tumors than broad-band UVB through the formation of cyclobutane pyrimidine dimer. *J Invest Dermatol*. Vol.127, No.12, (December 2007), pp2865-2871.

Lee, AY.; Kim, NH.; Choi, WI. & Youm, YH. (2005). Less keratinocyte-derived factors related to more keratinocyte apoptosis in depigmented than normally pigmented suction-blistered epidermis may cause passive melanocyte death in vitiligo. *J Invest Dermatol*. Vol.124, No.5, (May 2005), pp976-983.

Lowney, YW.; Ruby, MV.; Wester, RC.; Schoof, RA.; Holm, SE.; Hui, XY.; Barbadillo, S. & Maibach, HI. (2005). Percutaneous absorption of arsenic from environmental media. *Toxicol Ind Health*. Vol.21, No.1-2, (March 2005), pp1-14.

Majid, I. (2010). Topical placental extract: does it increase the efficacy of narrowband UVB therapy in vitiligo? *Indian J Dermatol Venereol Leprol*. Vol.76, No.3, (May 2010), pp 254-258.

Middelkamp-Hup, MA.; Bos, JD.; Rius-Diazm F.; Gonzalez, S. & Westerhof, W. Treatment of vitiligo vulgaris with narrow-band UVB and oral Polypodium leucotomos extract: a randomized double-blind placebo-controlled study. *J Eur Acad Dermatol Venereol.* Vol.21, No.7, (August 2007), pp942-950.

Mofty, ME.; Zaher, H.; Esmat, S.; Youssef, R.; Shahin, Z.; Bassioni, D. & Enani, GE. (2001). PUVA and PUVB in vitiligo--are they equally effective? *Photodermatol Photoimmunol Photomed.* Vol.17, No.4, (August 2001), pp159-163.

Namazi, MR. & Chee Leok, GO. (2009). Vitiligo and diet: a theoretical molecular approach with practical implications. *Indian J Dermatol Venereol Leprol.* Vol.75, No.2, (March 2009), pp116-118.

Park, SD.; Lee, SW.; Chun, JH. & Cha, SH. (2000). Clinical features of 31 patients with systemic contact dermatitis due to the ingestion of Rhus (lacquer). *Br J Dermatol.* 2000 May;142(5):937-42.

Patel, DC.; Evans, AV.& Hawk, JL. (2002). Topical pseudocatalase mousse and narrowband UVB phototherapy is not effective for vitiligo: an open, single-centre study. *Clin Exp Dermatol.* Vol.27, No.8, (November 2002), pp641-644.

Parsad, D.; Pandhi, R. & Juneja, A. (2003). Effectiveness of oral Ginkgo biloba in treating limited, slowly spreading vitiligo. *Clin Exp Dermatol.* Vol.28, No.3, (May 2003), pp285-287.

Pires, MC.; Martins, JM.; Montealegre, F. & Gatti, FR. (2010). Vitiligo after diphencyprone for alopecia areata. *Dermatol Res Pract.* Vol. 2010, (May 2010), p171265.

Rajatanavin, N.; Suwanachote, S. & Kulkollakarn, S. (2008). Dihydroxyacetone: a safe camouflaging option in vitiligo. *Int J Dermatol.* Vol.47, No.4, (April 2008), pp402-406.

Ravish, K. (August 2011). Vitiligo diet, *In: Ayurhealthline, 22,08,2011, Available from* http://www.ayurhealthline.com/Vitiligo-Diet.html

Rosenbach, T.; Wellenreuther, U.; Nurnberger, F. & Czarnetzki, BM. (1993). Treatment of vitiligo with phenylalanine and UV-A. *Hautarzt.* Vol.44, No.4, (July 1993), pp208-209.

Saper, RB.; Kales, SN.; Paquin, J.; Burns, MJ.; Eisenberg, DM.; Davis, RB. & Phillips, RS. (2004). Heavy metal content of ayurvedic herbal medicine products. *JAMA.* Vol.292, No.23, (December 2004), pp2868-2873.

Sarveswari, KN. (2010). Cosmetic camouflage in vitiligo. *Indian J Dermatol.* Vol.55, No.3, (July 2010), pp211-214.

Schallreuter, KU.; Wood, JM.; Lemke, KR. & Levenig, C. (1995). Treatment of vitiligo with a topical application of pseudocatalase and calcium in combination with short-term UVB exposure: a case study on 33 patients. *Dermatology.* Vol.190, No.3, (March 1995), pp223 -229.

Schallreuter, KU.; Moore, J.; Wood, JM.; Beazley, WD.; Gaze, DC.; Tobin, DJ.; Marshall, HS.; Panske, A.; Panzig, E. & Hibberts, NA. (1999). In vivo and in vitro evidence for hydrogen peroxide (H2O2) accumulation in the epidermis of patients with vitiligo and its successful removal by a UVB-activated pseudocatalase. *J Investig Dermatol Symp Proc.* Vol.4, No.1, (September 1999), pp91-96.

Schallreuter, KU.; Moore, J.; Wood, JM.; Beazley, WD.; Peters, EM.; Marles, LK.; Behrens-Williams, SC.; Dummer, R.; Blau, N. & Thöny, B. (2001). Epidermal H_2O_2 accumulation alters tetrahydrobiopterin (6BH4) recycling in vitiligo: identification of a general mechanism in regulation of all 6BH4-dependent processes? *J Invest Dermatol.* Vol.116, No.1, (January 2001), pp167-174.

Schallreuter, KU & Rokos, H. (2005). Vitix-a new treatment for vitiligo? *Int J Dermatol.* Vol.44, No.11, (November 2005), pp969-970.

Serrano, G.; Lorente, M.; Reyes, M.; Millan, F.; Lloret, A; Melendez, J.; Navarro, M. & Navarro, M. (2009). Photodynamic therapy with low-strength ALA, repeated applications and short contact periods (40-60 minutes) in acne, photoaging and vitiligo. *J Drugs Dermatol*. Vol.8, No.6, (June 2009), pp562-568.

Sharma, AD. (2007). Relationship between nickel allergy and diet. *Indian J Dermatol Venereol Leprol*. Vol.73, No.5, (September 2007), pp307-312.

Shin, JU.; Roh, MR. & Lee, JH. (2010. Vitiligo following intense pulsed light treatment. *J Dermatol*. Vol.37, No.7, (July 2010), pp674-676.

Siddiqui, AH.; Stolk, LM.; Bhaggoe, R.; Hu, R.; Schutgens, RB. & Westerhof, W. (1994). L-phenylalanine and UVA irradiation in the treatment of vitiligo. *Dermatology*. Vol.188, No.3, (March 1994), pp215-218.

Simopoulos, AP. (2002). Omega-3 fatty acids in inflammation and autoimmune diseases. *J Am Coll Nutr*. Vol.21, No.6, (December 2002), pp495-505.

Singh, AK. & Karki, D. (2010). Micropigmentation: tattooing for the treatment of lip vitiligo. *J Plast Reconstr Aesthet Surg*. Vol.63, No.6, (June 2010), pp988-991.

Srivastava, RK. (August, 2011). *Vitiligo (leukoderma) Ayurvedic treatment*. 22/08/2011, Availble from http://ayurveda-foryou.com/treat/leucoderma.html .

Suga, Y.; Ikejima, A.; Matsuba, S. & Ogawa, H. (2002). Medical pearl: DHA application for camouflaging segmental vitiligo and piebald lesions. *J Am Acad Dermatol*. Vol.47, No.3, (September 2002), pp436-438.

Szczurko, O.; Shear, N.; Taddio, A. & Boon, H. (2011). Ginkgo biloba for the treatment of vitilgo vulgaris: an open label pilot clinical trial. *BMC Complement Altern Med*. Vol.11, (March 2011), p21.

Spritz, RA. (2011). Recent progress in the genetics of generalized vitiligo. *J Genet Genomics*. Vol.38, No.7, (July 2011), pp271-278.

Taïeb, A. & Picardo, M. (2009). Clinical practice. Vitiligo. *N Engl J Med*. Vol.362, No.2, (January 2009), pp160-169.

Tanioka, M. & Miyachi, Y. (2008). Waterproof camouflage for vitiligo of the face using Cavilon 3M as a spray. *Eur J Dermatol*. Vol.18, No.1, (January 2008), pp93-94.

Tanioka, M. & Miyachi, Y. (2009). Camouflage for vitiligo. *Dermatol Ther*. Vol.22, No.1, (January 2009), pp90-93.

Tanioka, M.; Yamamoto, Y.; Kato, M. & Miyachi, Y. (2010). Camouflage for patients with vitiligo vulgaris improved their quality of life. *J Cosmet Dermatol*. Vol.9, No.1, (March 2010), pp72-75.

Teschke, R. & Bahre, R. (2009). Severe hepatotoxicity by Indian Ayurvedic herbal products: a structured causality assessment. *Ann Hepatol*. Vol.8, No.3, (July 2009), pp258-266.

Vanherweghem, JL. ; Depierreux, M. ; Tielemans, C. ; Abramowicz, D. ; Dratwa, M. ; Jadoul, M. ; Richard, C. *et al*. (1993). Rapidly progressive interstitial renal fibrosis in young women: association with slimming regimen including Chinese herbs. *Lancet*. Vol.341, No.8842, (February 1993), pp387-391.

Yuksel, EP.; Aydin, F.; Senturk, N.; Canturk, T. & Turanli, AY. (2009). Comparison of the efficacy of narrow band ultraviolet B and narrow band ultraviolet B plus topical catalase-superoxide dismutase treatment in vitiligo patients. *Eur J Dermatol*. Vol.19, No.4, (July 2009), pp341-344.